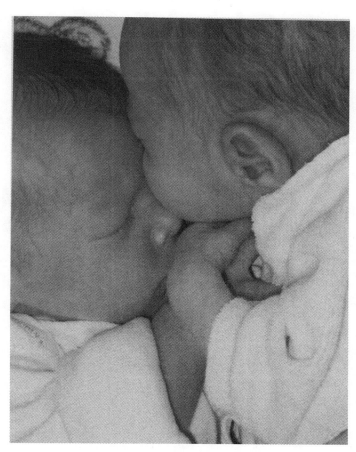

. . . A Mystical Journey

Whose Illness is it Anyway?

A Mystical Journey to Wellness

by

Marilyn Segal and Carolyn Cohen

Whose Illness is it Anyway

Published by Twin-Lynn, Inc.
Atlanta, Georgia
Printed in the United States of America
ISBN Nol 0-964040350-14

Cover Photograpy and Inside photography by Lisa Delvin
Cover Design by DiBona Design, Atlanta, Georgia.
Printing Coordination by TruPrint, Atlanta, Georgia

5 4 3 2 1

Also by Marilyn Segal:
The Heart Speaks

Also by Carolyn Cohen:
Precious Reflections

We dedicate our book to
the late Dr. Norman Cousins
and our mother,
Janet Berman Levine

Write First — Speak Later

the late Dr. Norman Cousins

Table of Contents

Acknowledgements

First and most importantly, we want to thank God for reaching out to us in our darkest times and gently guiding us to find our truths. We want to thank our angels, both here and on Earth, for being there for us. It's been fun working with them and involving them in our every day life.

There have been so many people who took their time to help us bring this book to fruition. A big thanks to my husband, Terry, for all his love and support. He truly is my biggest fan. Carolyn and I both thank Mike, Carolyn's husband for supporting and loving her in her darkest times.

A special thanks to Nancy Neman and Kathy Curry. Nancy, a dear friend of ours, helped bring enthusiasm and freshness to our project. She helped us bring form to it. Kathy Curry had the insight and creativity to literally sit down with us, word by word, until completion. Without them this book would probably still be an unfulfilled dream. Our deepest gratitude.

Our deepest appreciation to Pat DiBona, our graphic designer, for envisioning the final design. And thank you, Lisa Devlin, our photographer, for capturing our spirit in our photographs. Thank you to all those who helped along the way proofing, editing, rereading: Phyllis Mueller, the late Steve Nelson, Jim Kelton, Tony Markham, Sue Serrins, Bob Peace, Mary Beth

Schommer, Patty Rampone, Suzi Brozman and Joan Schwartz.

      We want to thank Eleanor Cousins who earlier in our writing, encouraged us to write the ending so we'd have an end point in sight. We are grateful to have been a bridge for her and her late husband, Norman.

      We want to thank Laurz Segal, Marilyn's sister-in-law, for introducing us to California clients: Jackie Banchik, Diana Davidow, Sherri Pine, Ina Lewis, Toni Karp, Marlene Bronson, Sarah & Joel Piehl and Toby Rothman. Not only were they our teachers, they were our jump-start to the work we do today.

      A big, big thank you to Charles & Nicole Kaplan who blessed us with a picture of their twins, Isabel & Lily, which we used in the front of the book. And a final thank you to our family and friends who love and support us always, and to Ruby Segal, Marilyn's mother-in-law, who made room in her heart not only for us but for all our sisters.

Editorial Note

By Nancy Flemming Neman

In this "cosmic millennium age" of year 2000, it is no longer unusual to come across articles in the newspaper or hear a friend or stranger discuss angels, telepathy, kinesthetic energy, vortexes, crystals, healing hands and a variety of other so-called "new age" topics. The reactions that I have observed to all this range from whole-hearted agreement to debate about whose method is better to "Doubting Thomas's" to outright eye-rolling.

This is one of many reasons why I urge you to choose this book to take home with you. Although there are numerous "charlatans", false prophets, greedy seers and just plain old crackpot Amercanized distorters of some very old and mystical topics, the authors of this book, twin sisters Carolyn and Marilyn Levine, are definitely, positively, and absolutely for real. What they say in this book is also for real; on the level of life changing words, ideas, and most of all, spirit.

I had the good fortune to meet Carolyn and Marilyn Levine many years ago in grade school, so that means I have known them for a long time. I know that they started out just like we all did…with our own dramas and traumas (as they say so eloquently)…just like the rest of us. Through jr. high school, when we were discovering boys and were mostly governed by hormones, they were C students like the rest of us. In jr. high and high school, their names weren't on the "Most Likely To Succeed" yearbook list. They were just Carolyn and Marilyn, the twins, who were liked by all and loved by their close friends. They gave of themselves even back then, through their loving, generous and compassionate spirits. It surprised me while editing this book that during our younger years they had gone through so much pain; as their wonderful senses of humor and fun-loving ways concealed that painful trauma from all their friends. We spent a lot of time together, too—classes, after school activities, week-ends, slumber parties—all the typical things that close friends do.

What I am trying to say here is that Marilyn and Carolyn were, and are, *real* people just like you. They haven't always had, or rather used, their current awesome, unbelievable, God-inspired "powers". They have been touched by God; by the positive force from our universe. It only takes the smallest moment to realize this in the deepest part of your being when you talk with them, read what they have written, attend one of their seminars or healings, or just be around them. Carolyn even went so far as to experience the "other side" personally in her near death experience. Marilyn did, too, although the "other side" came to her through her contacts right here in her life experiences.

As you will see in this book, their experiences are awe-inspiring and can touch you, too. Plus, it is an enjoyable and fascinating read.

First, their stories are spellbinding. Then, the mystery of what in the world is going to happen next is an absolute page-turner. Then, the insights and realizations that they share with you as a result of what they experienced and learned can make your being sing with joy. If you ever do yourself a favor, meet Carolyn and Marilyn and read this book.

When I finished editing this book, I missed reading it so much. It was my friend, my guide, my teacher, and it can be yours, too. It is not only their story, it is the positive force of the universe speaking through them and their experiences.

Through their story, you can meet with God.

Part I

Two by Two
A Mystical Journey to Wellness

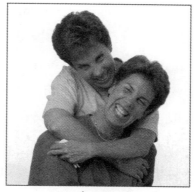

Marilyn & Carolyn

Whose Illness is it Anyway ?

*W*hose **Illness is It Anyway** is a story about a journey that we, as identical twins, took together in our struggle with our life's challenges through illness. We each played a vital role in one another's well being. I, Marilyn, was stuck with debilitating back pain for twenty-seven years and had an instantaneous healing. The question that ultimately led us to our freedom was, "Why wasn't Carolyn freed at the same time?"

Three months later, in a near death experience, Carolyn did at last let go of her symptom. It was from there that we realized there is a grand rhythm and mystery to life that we had previously not understood. We recognized that if we had been set free at the same time, we wouldn't have gone on to search for the mysteries life was unfolding for us to share.

What we have learned is, although everyone has his or her own story with its unique struggles and challenges, traumas and dramas, there is hope for your truths to emerge so your happiness can step out to dance with you, too. We feel this happened to us, as twins, so we could share with you the possibility that when you are "stuck," it is time to begin your own detective work. Look for outside clues as to who (or what) might be entangled in your life and causing you harm. We have found through working with others, that this can happen not only to twins, but also with mother and daughter, father and son, husband and wife, your best friend or even with someone who is deceased. God has a plan on how He wants to wake each of us up to realize how we all are connected to everything. He wants us to know that by learning to help ourselves, we learn how to help others. We joke about it now, but we couldn't believe that the missing ingredient to our well being was our connection to God. Our religious interpretation about God had been that God was outside of us and unreachable.

It wasn't until we made that personal connection with God, each individually and together, that our voids were finally filled.

Instead of telling you details about our lives and our upbringing, we find it more rewarding to share our "presence" with you. The insights we have gathered from our adventures and the intuition that we developed led us to more possibilities. From these insights Carolyn and I will take you back into those powerful six months that left us in awe of our spiritual path. The layout for this book will be a little different. We will start with our third wake-up call and move back in time. I, (Marilyn) feel that Dr. Norman Cousins was the necessary catalyst for me/us to get serious and write about our journey. Since we are two people, having similar experiences, we have decided to use different fonts. I, Marilyn, will be the main voice in this book, speaking in a slanted font. Carolyn will be interjecting in a straight up and down font.

Perhaps now would be a good time to ask you to sit back, take off your shoes, and get comfortable so you, too, can begin a similar journey. Begin by asking your own questions to life's "what-if's." Through our discovery, we would like to invite you to start uncovering the real you and discover your own hidden talents. To awaken your consciousness and begin blessing this world with your beauty. To awaken your mind and connect to the omnipresence in all things.

To learn how to reach for an angel when you need one most and open your heart to the Divine.

Marilyn
&
Carolyn

Early Saturday morning, the telephone rang. I awoke from a deep sleep.

"Did you see the late news last night?" the disembodied voice said. I felt I was dreaming.

"No," I said, still groggy from sleep.

"Norman Cousins died yesterday."

I bolted upright, trembling as chills poured through my body.

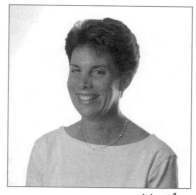

Marilyn

Marilyn's Meeting with Norman Cousins
Wake Up Call Number Three

*I*t was November 1990 when I received my third wake-up call in six months. Answers seemed to find their way to me in the most unexpected circumstances. I was visiting my sister-in-law, Laurz, in Los Angeles. A friend of hers, Diana, was attending a fund-raiser for the John Wayne Cancer Auxiliary. Norman Cousins was to be their guest speaker. I had already read Dr. Cousins' book, **Anatomy of An Illness**. On that day, he was to present his new book, **Biology of Hope**. Naturally I wanted to attend, because he was "right up my alley" and had knowledge for which I was hungry.

I remember the day well. It was Wednesday, November 28th. The room was huge, enhanced by its glitzy lights and crystal. I remember my feelings vividly, the energy from the room was exhilarating. People were hustling and bustling with excitement to find their seats. About nine hundred people filled the room.

When Dr. Cousins was introduced, he was handsomely applauded. I don't remember his speech but I do remember that I felt he was speaking directly to me. As the words flowed from his mouth, I knew I must speak to this man. He spoke for about thirty or forty minutes. His voice seemed weak to me, but oh, how powerful were his words!

After his speech, I felt a strong urge to speak to him privately. This little voice inside my head told me to go speak with him and an invisible hand literally pushed me in his direction. I felt awkward, because this behavior was so unlike me.

I thought to myself, "If I do introduce myself, what will I say?" Everything happened so fast, and before I knew it I was directly in front of Dr. Cousins. I felt extremely nervous as I introduced myself. I blurted out my question, "If a person is sick, and that person has an identical twin, should both of them be seen by the doctor?"

I didn't think my question made any sense at the time, but I knew if anybody would understand it would be him. My hunch was that he would understand.

Immediately after hearing my question, Dr. Cousins gave an odd sort of smile and asked if I could see him in his office. WOW! I expected an answer, not an invitation. I told him I was to be in Los Angeles for only a few more days. He said that would not be a problem. He gave me his number and asked that I call his assistant, Barbara, to set up an appointment.

I was elated! The moment I returned to Laurz's apartment I made that call, only to be told there were no available appointments for that week. I left the number where I could be reached. I felt disappointed, but somewhere in my heart I knew I was supposed to see this man and I knew an appointment would come available.

The next day, I got a call from Barbara that someone had canceled and a time slot was available. It was for Friday, November 30, 1990. It exhilarated me to think that I was going to see Dr. Cousins. I wondered what I had said to him that had triggered this invitation.

Friday arrived quickly. It was a beautiful sunny California day; I felt so alive. Terry, my husband, had come out the previous night for business and we were staying at the J. W. Marriott on Avenue of the Stars. Laurz was to pick me up and take me to Dr. Cousins' office at UCLA. I wanted to look perfect and say the right things without coming across as a goof-ball. Needless to say, I was scared, anxious and excited all at the same time.

Three o'clock rolled around and before I knew it I was inside Dr. Cousins' office. I reminded myself to breathe and to talk slowly. My mind had a rapid pace of talking and I often stumbled over words. It was important that I clearly communicate my findings to Dr. Cousins so that I might inquire about what possible direction to take. As I walked into his office, he rose from his chair to shake my hand. We simultaneously thanked each other for being there. He invited me to take a seat on his couch while he sat down at his desk. I asked him why he had invited me to see him.

He replied, "You aroused my curiosity."

That was my cue to pour out my findings. I began rapidly talking about my twin sister and her illness, and how we had been intertwined in each other's illnesses. I told him we had identified the so-called mystical connection between us and the adventure we had been on, including the reappearance of our deceased mother. I told him about Carolyn's near-death experience and how peaceful death really is.

Dr. Cousins came out from behind his desk and sat down next to me on the couch. He took my hand into his and just held it. I realized that he thought I had said Carolyn had died. I corrected myself and said that she had lived. Nevertheless, he continued to hold my hand. (A thought appeared in my head, 'Was he making a pass at me?' I watched for any signs.) Our conversation continued and all he could do was tell me to write about all of this, including about my mother. He thought it so fascinating. He kept repeating the words, "Write first, then speak." About this time I saw a gray haze encompassing his body but at the time I did not have the knowledge of what "that" was. I had the definite feeling that Dr. Cousins was supposed to help me do something.

Barbara came into the room and quietly told him his next appointment was running a little late. All I could hear was that it was in a nearby hotel. I knew our time was almost up and wondered what had been accomplished by our meeting. Just like at the luncheon two days before, his voice was weak but it amazed me how strong and powerful his words were. Before I left, Dr. Cousins asked to see my family pictures. He commented that Carolyn's husband, Mike, looked like a rabbi. In some sort of an odd way, I felt connected to Dr. Cousins—as if I had known him my whole life. He got up from the couch and I knew it was time to say good-bye. He looked at me and asked for a small favor. He asked if he could have a hug.

"Of course," I smiled. "I was going to give you one anyway."

As we embraced, you could have knocked us both out of the room with our energy exchange, almost as if a tidal wave had pushed us off balance. We laughed about that hug and said we had never experienced anything like it before.

I thanked him for seeing me and before walking out the door, I asked, "Would you consider helping me explore my connection with Carolyn and my mother? Or could you help point me in the direction I might need to go with this type of information?"

He said he would give it some thought and told me to leave my name, phone *number and address with Barbara.*

I left the information with Barbara and before leaving the office I asked her, "Is he feeling all right?" She said he had been feeling a little tired but that was all.

I left the office and stopped at a phone across the hall. I called Laurz to tell her I was ready to be picked up. Suddenly all the enthusiasm I felt thirty minutes before drained out of me. I wondered what had happened between the two of us. I laughed at myself for thinking that Dr. Cousins had been trying to make a pass at me, but a girl has to be cautious these days. For the past few months I had been getting some intuitive hunches that usually proved significant. I knew Dr. Cousins was supposed to help me do something, but what?

Laurz couldn't pick me up for another hour, so I found a quiet place to sit down and think. By this time my body felt chilled and very cold. I didn't understand why I felt physically cold and emotionally drained; it was a warm, sunny California day. I felt as if the life force had been sucked out of me. As I sat waiting, I thought about my meeting with Dr. Cousins. I had already started writing my memoirs the year before. I wondered what Dr.Cousins meant when he said, "Write first, then speak."

Was I supposed to continue writing about Carolyn's and my journey comparing each of us to the other? Was I supposed to write about my mother's sudden reappearance in this physical plane? Was I supposed to write about Carolyn's near-death experience and the peacefulness of the thereafter? I looked at my watch; it was 5:13 p.m. I wondered where Laurz was. Suddenly I became even colder. I heard the distinctive honk from Laurz' car; I jumped up and hurried to get in. I was happy to be going back to her place.

After his last meeting, Terry checked out of the hotel and headed off to meet us back at Laurz's, where we would stay the weekend. We had plans to go out that night. All I wanted was a hot drink, a good meal, a warm bath, and a good night's sleep.

Laurz had arranged for me to meet a friend of hers, Sherri, the next morning, who had battled and survived ovarian cancer. Laurz thought that Sherri and I would have a lot to talk about.

We canceled our plans that night. Laurz and Terry did something without me. After dinner, I had my warm shower and went to bed. But before going to bed, I told both Laurz and Terry, "I met Norman Cousins today for a reason. I don't know for what, but I'll find out in the morning."

Early the next morning we were awakened by a phone call from Diana, the woman who had invited me to the Norman Cousins luncheon. She told us that Norman Cousins had died. Chills and more chills radiated throughout my body.

My first question was, "Do you know what happened and at what time he died?"

Laurz went out to get the morning paper. All the information was there except the time. I found out later that Dr. Cousins died around 5:13—that was the time I felt heavy chills pour through my body.

I got ready to meet Laurz' friend, Sherri. Sherri must have been a God-send. She explained to me that Norman Cousins had sought me out in the crowd as much as I had sought him. I had never heard this kind of talk or explanation before. It was all so new to me. Sherri explained that I must have provided the answer or the connection for Norman Cousins to feel safe enough to leave.

The events that transpired from there until my writing about my meeting with Norman Cousins helped explain what had happened in my own mother's transformation into death. I discovered that these "subtle energies" left behind by the person leaving could become quite transforming for the people still on this physical plane. In my own case with my mother, I felt like an abandoned fawn, stuck and afraid to move. My experience with Norman Cousins became the bridge from my past pains into my new life awareness. His passing helped explain some of my own pains. Sherri explained that I must have been a piece of Dr. Cousins' puzzle, too—so many things happen at so many levels—all entwined with each other. I asked her where she had received her knowledge and she said it happened in her own healing process with cancer. She felt as if she had gone to a place "beyond" to heal.

Sherri became one of my mentors that day, and to this day she is still my friend. She has continued to help me find answers and explanations to events I experience by filling in the gaps I miss. We are all each other's teachers. We are all students. We all are mirrors for each other, reflecting to one another what needs attention and what needs to be healed in our deepest levels of existence.

That's when I began entertaining the possibility that I had created all my pains through my thoughts and bottled up emotions. Was it possible that my thoughts were the missing equation and silent partner to all my pains? Was it possible that Carolyn had been reflecting back to me my blocked emotions? What better way to see your own reflection than through a personal mirror—your twin?

The days that I had contact with Norman Cousins were a part of my own puzzle. Even though he had appeared weak, his thoughts were extremely strong. I wondered if I had been hearing other people's thoughts as well. Little did I know, I was opening a very major door of communication with the unspoken word. I was aware that Carolyn and I had telepathic communication. Had I been conversing with others in the same way, but beyond my awareness? Maybe that was the reason for my confusion around communication. I sensed one form of communication but heard another, and words and actions didn't match.

Was this form of communication any different than the one I had been learning from my mother? Was this form of communication any different than the one I used to talk with God? I had shared with Dr. Cousins the secret communication skills I had developed. Little did I know that I was keeping that door of communication open to Dr. Cousins.

What I had discovered was that communication doesn't have to be any different with someone who has passed over. The only difference is the fear of not knowing how to keep that communication open. We each have our own experiences. My initial meeting with Norman Cousins was in the physical form. The communication then changed into spirit form (Remember the chills I had? The chills was spirit talking.) That experience allowed me to remember what had happened to me the night my mother died and freed me from fearing those feelings anymore. Those similar feelings had been my mother's spirit passing through me, except then I didn't want to let her go. Carolyn and I had both been holding onto her.

Meeting Dr. Cousins was truly a blessing. As the days and the months passed by, I received more confirmations.

Lets Take a Walk

Upon returning to Atlanta from the California trip, I came down with a horrendous cold. My body had not yet chilled out. I felt stiff and I ached. My nose ran continuously for the next twenty-four hours, and I couldn't keep enough tissues on hand. I knew that this cold had something to do with Dr. Cousins.

The next morning, intuitively I knew that writing about my experience would clear up my runny nose. I furiously began writing about our meeting. I must have written for two-and-a-half hours when I decided to take a break and go for a walk. It was cold outside but the sun was bright, so I bundled up and went out for my walk. I noticed my nose was no longer running. I sighed deeply and smiled. I knew contact had been made. I needed to wait for Dr. Cousins' reply, in whatever form he chose.

During my healing process, one of my rituals was to meditate. I had always thought that meditation was weird, but that was because I didn't understand its purpose. I had always talked to God, even before my wake-up calls. I called it "my own personal contact with God" to negotiate with the pain in my body. I would tell God how I planned to handle the pain from my end, and could He do His part. Meditation was a time for me to be quiet and listen to God. Meditation became a daily habit to quiet myself and to connect with God and all of my wonderful surroundings.

Shortly after my meeting with Norman Cousins, I was meditating. I experienced a vibration in my body; like an intense hug or cradling. The vibration reminded me of my visit with the late Dr. Cousins. I wondered if I was making all if this up. During this meditation, Dr. Cousins talked with me in thought forms. His thought forms were as strong to me as the day I had met with him. I made notes on what he was telling me. Over the next several months, I found myself getting up at 3:00 a.m. to record on paper the thought forms I felt I was sharing with Norman Cousins. I wrote about things I had never before thought about. Also, when I played a certain kind of piano music, I could feel my body rock with "his" familiar vibration.

During a later meditation, Dr. Cousins told me, in thought form, his wife would be contacting me and gave me the numbers 9 and 20. I had no clue as to what that meant. Was it a time? Was it a date? It was February, so it must have meant a time. My next thoughts were, "She doesn't even know me. How's this going to happen?"

I found that when you ask questions, the universe will provide the answers—in the universe's time frame. Many months went by. It was late summer and I was attending a metaphysical fair in Atlanta. I passed by some books and the book that caught my eye was **Celebration of Life** by Norman Cousins. I bought the book, again, out of curiosity. It was a collection of essays that had not been published until after his death.

In it, I found some of the same information I had been writing about for so many months. It was my confirmation that I was communicating with the late Dr. Cousins. Then in September, I had another confirmation. It was a Friday afternoon. I felt an extremely strong connection to Mrs, Cousins. I didn't know why; I had not met her yet. The thoughts soon passed. On Monday I got a letter dated 9/20—those were the numbers I recieved from Dr. Cousins while meditating months earlier. I smiled and looked up to the Universe and Dr. Cousins to give my, "Thanks!"

On my next visit to California I was compelled to call Mrs. Cousins. She agreed to meet me, a complete stranger. I nervously told her on the phone that I was the last appointment her husband had before his death.

I met with her the next day in a little coffee shop on Montana Avenue in Santa Monica. Again, I got another confirmation. I found out that the last scheduled appointment with Dr. Cousins the day of his death had been with a pianist. He, too, played piano by ear.

As strange as it was, I showed Mrs. Cousins my writings. She was amazed at the similarities. We talked for about an hour and a half, until she needed to get home to let her dog out. I joked and inquisitively asked, "Is your dog's name Charlie?" She looked at me with astonishment and politely smiled with the reply, "Yes." Before she left, she invited me to come to her house the following day. I agreed. Now I had all this new information. What was I to do with it? I kept hearing Dr. Cousins' words, "Write first, then speak."

All of us have our own stories and wake-up calls. My meeting with Norman Cousins put a new door in front of me to open. I went through this door into the abyss, much like I had experiences with Carolyn. Dr. Cousins was the confirmation to let me know that my answers are my truths and no one else can find them for me. He was the bridge to let me know that the still, quiet voice inside was really God.

Since my meeting with the late Dr. Cousins, life has been nothing short of one continuous adventure. So many doors and possibilities have presented themselves. After several years of writing, I have finally come to the conclusion that I must share my exciting adventure with others. I must share this knowledge that I keep receiving. It is my gift.

Ants work piece-by-piece, bringing crumbs back to the nest until their mound is noticeable to those who come onto its path. That is our hope for those who read this work. If our writings, our journey, can spark an "ah-ha" in your life, to set you onto your own inner discovery of personal truths, this will be the greatest gift we can give as fellow sparks of God's creation. May God be with you.

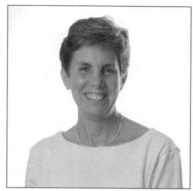

Carolyn

Carolyn's Near-Death Experience
Wake Up Call No. 2-Three Months Earlier

*I*t was in August of 1990 when my twin sister, Carolyn, died--or at least had a "near-death experience". She said she died. I don't know if it is more accurate to say that she died and then came back, or if she just came close to dying. It all amounts to the same thing. First you're here, then you're not, and then you're back again.

This horrifying episode began innocently enough on a Friday evening. Terry and I had just sold our condo and were preparing to move into our first house. The condo was packed with boxes waiting for our move. We were enjoying dinner with my twin and her husband, Mike, at their home. My younger sister, Debra, and her friend, Beth, were in from New York for the weekend. It was late August and the heat and humidity were stifling. It had been one of those sticky, sauna days for which Atlanta summers are famous. Carolyn had been suffering with lower back pain all day and had even taken a few extra aspirins with codeine. After dinner, I worked with Carolyn demonstrating a technique I used to relieve some of my pains.

As Carolyn lay on the floor trying to stretch out the muscles around her pelvic girdle, I said, "You know, this pain, these symptoms, look like the pain I used to have. When I wore my back brace, I used to feel like this all the time." Jokingly, I added, "Maybe you get to share some of my pain."

"I don't care whose symptoms these are, just get them out of me. I just want to get comfortable. I can't go into the weekend with this excruciating back pain combined with one of my coughing attacks."

It seemed like the words had barely left her mouth when she began to cough— a dry, chronic cough that had afflicted her for years, often requiring hospitalization. That cough had forced dramatic and profound changes in my sister's life.

It was no ordinary cough; it had taken over my life. It was much like a hiccup that would not stop. It sounded like guttural noises coming from deep within my chest and throat. It came without warning, lasting one to three hours, but never longer. It appeared at least two times a day and sometimes three. And always, like a perverse alarm clock, it would wake me up at three a.m. It stifled my breath, forced incontinence and vomiting to the point of broken ribs. Sweat would gush from every pore on my body. My neck and shoulders would tense up to brace my body as I coughed and coughed and threw up. One good result was that my stomach was as tight as a washboard from the sit-up crunches I did during the coughing spells; which struck me as an odious way to achieve a girlhood dream. Strangely enough, when the "attack" was over it was like it had never happened. In another time I would have been exorcised for demonic possession, but in our enlightened age, the doctors simply did not know what to do for these violent attacks so devastating to me. They gave me a broad assortment of paraphernalia to keep at my bedside in case of emergencies. Every night as I lay in bed, I had unusual company: an oxygen tank, a bronchodilator machine, adrenaline, steroids, inhalers, a trash can and lots of Kleenex. Depending on how strenuous the coughs were, they sometimes made my throat passage so swollen I could not take in air.

About eight months into these episodes, during an x-ray exam, the radiologist found a small growth on my esophagus. When he pushed on the lump, I began to cough hysterically. We thought we had found the reason for this strange cough.

I met the thoracic surgeon and within a few days I was under his knife. Prior to the surgery, I told him I didn't want any negative talk during the operation, unaware at this time how powerful words are, even when you are not conscious of what is being said. He agreed. After surgery, he told me he had removed a tumor as large as a lemon from my trachea, which had been wrapped around my vocal cords. The surgery was successful from an operative point, and we were all optimistic that we had at last found the answer. … Wrong!

Within a week the cough started to return. It began gradually, but within a month it was full blown. "It's ba-a-a-ck" -but in a strange way it was different. My voice was weakened by the surgery. I couldn't speak very loudly and if I talked even for a short period of time, it sent me into one of my coughing attacks.

I sought out ear, nose, and throat doctors all over the city, getting opinion after opinion. They discovered that one vocal cord had been paralyzed from the surgery and recommended that I not do anything for at least a year to see how the vocal cord repaired itself.

Two months after surgery I encouraged my pulmonary doctor to put me back into the hospital for more tests. Once again I was numbed up and probed. The test results reported the same: "aggravated airways, etiology unknown". I was tired. I needed a break from this "cough monster." I encouraged the pulmonologist to try steroids because in the past small doses had provided short-term relief. This time the doctor planned to experiment with higher dosages, hopefully knocking out the cough altogether.

By the third day of this treatment, I regained my taste and smell. I remembered that just before I lost these senses, I had become hypersensitive to smells. It was the spring of 1988, and everything blooming became acutely intensified and so overwhelming that I literally became sick to my stomach. I was so overwhelmed with all the fragrances that my body automatically began to protect me by simply turning off my senses of taste and smell. These two senses had been gone for about six months and with their return, I suddenly realized I had become hypersensitive to my environment.

Although I had many questions about this sudden hypersensitivity, they were not to be answered until much later.

The events from that Friday night continue.

Carolyn got up from the floor, where I was working with her, to go upstairs to get her breathing machine. I motioned to Terry that I thought it was time for us to go home, but Mike yelled to Terry from the upstairs bedroom to come and help carry down the oxygen tank. That meant we were on our way to the hospital.

I remember walking upstairs to get my breathing machine. Mike followed me upstairs to get my oxygen and began to load a syringe with adrenaline. He later told me that he knew something was wrong because I was very calm. I had recently learned how to meditate. So my first thought was, "Oh, meditation must be working. I do feel peaceful amidst all this chaos." Somehow or somewhere I could feel my spirit and my body begin to detach.

I yelled to Mike, "Get the other breathing machine, this one is not working right." That alerted Mike even more because the other breathing machine was even harder to use. Mike gave me a shot of adrenaline, but it didn't work like it usually did.

"I'm taking you to the hospital," he said.

I would usually resist, but this night, still feeling very peaceful, I accepted his directive. Time seemed to slow down. I began to see my family buzzing around me in order to bring cohesiveness into all this drama. Mike called downstairs for Terry's assistance. My first thought as I began to walk down the hall was, "How do people walk in these dense bodies?" Mike guided me down the stairs, while Terry carried my oxygen tank and Marilyn followed from behind. Outside, it was a typical muggy evening. I wondered how people breathed in this dense air.

We put Carolyn in the front seat of the van with her oxygen tank and I jumped in the back. Terry followed in our car.

"Load up another syringe of adrenaline," Mike said, struggling to keep the panic out of his voice.

We were only five minutes from the hospital; Mike was driving like a maniac to get us there. He wanted me to give Carolyn her shot but I felt uncomfortable doing so from the backseat, especially with the manner of his driving. He briefly stopped the car to administer the adrenaline himself. Everything was happening so fast. All the way to the hospital I heard a faint little voice in my head saying, "This is going to be close. This is going to be close."

When we finally arrived at the hospital we were greeted by a nurse who knew Mike and Carolyn because they were frequent visitors during Carolyn's breathing emergencies. She hustled Carolyn inside where the staff took over.

Mike followed them in and I waited for Terry. By the time we got inside, I was frantic. I knew for Carolyn's sake, I needed to take a deep breath to help calm me down. I didn't want to pass any "worrisome vibes" to her. I watched the doctors hook

Carolyn up to what looked like a hundred machines. She seemed consumed by them all, her body in convulsions while tubes ran from every direction.

I stood outside her room in front of a large window. Calmly, I began talking telepathically to Carolyn, telling her that if she would just let go of her cough, she could heal herself. That's when I saw something that resembled a mirage hovering over Carolyn's body, like steam rising from hot pavement. I had no idea what it was; however, the most ineffable peace entered my body, as I knew Carolyn's life was going to be turned around.

Without any mention as to what I had just seen, I said to Terry, "I'd better go call our family and tell them where we are and that everything is okay." Terry looked at me as if he had caught my vision of insight that everything was okay.

I left to make the call. When I returned, Terry took me aside and said, "You're not going to believe this, but Carolyn died and came back."

"I know," I said, "and she's not going to have that cough anymore;" as if it was just a matter of fact. The drama had lifted and we entered Carolyn's room where she excitedly began telling us all about her experience.

I interrupted her and said, "You're not going to have that cough anymore. I saw it leave." We didn't know it then, but I was feeling the physical effects from Carolyn's adrenaline. It felt as if I had had twenty cups of coffee zooming inside every *cell of my body. I was so excited to tell her about my vision that the words actually took over her space. (That's a twin-thing…never allowing the other one to fully have their own experience.)*

Carolyn pushed aside my bizarre comment and said that she was loaded up with steroids. Of course her cough was now under control.

As for my near-death experience and me, I definitely don't think that I had a "first-class ticket" to go to the light. I must have been in cargo. I was in a murky place with lots of spirits around. I vividly felt like I had to go to the bathroom, and asked "Excuse me, where is the restroom?" I heard lots of laughter and the spirits' replies.

"We don't go to the bathroom here," and they kept on laughing.

Then my deceased mother appeared. I didn't see her true physical form, I just knew her essence. From knowing that I drew a tremendous amount of comfort. She had been showing herself to me over the years, and more frequently during the past couple of months through my dreams and sometimes in a waking state. I was always happy to see her, and now I had the understanding as to "why" she had been showing herself to me.

As I lay fluttering my eyes in the emergency room, trying to come back or wake up or whatever you do after one of these experiences, I remember telling a nurse about my sensation of wanting to go to the bathroom.

"Lots of patients report that," she said.

My doctor told me that I had been admitted to the intensive care unit for overnight observation. He wrote on the orders, "Allergic to everything. Do not go near her. She will tell you what she needs." He said he would return early in the morning to release me, as he didn't want to keep me in the hospital any longer than necessary for fear I would catch something with my compromised immune system.

They moved me into a private room in the intensive care unit. A nurse was waiting to help get me situated. She gave me a hospital gown, and when I slipped into the bathroom to change I discovered that the feeling I had experienced about going to the bathroom had been real. I told the nurse about it but she didn't seem concerned. She acted like this happened a lot, and I'm sure it did, but it had never happened to me. I later learned that when someone dies, the body excretes all its fluids. This is what happened to me. I felt so embarrassed. I gave the nurse my soiled clothes, and never saw them again.

As I settled in my room, I remembered Debra had been visiting us from New York for the weekend. It dawned on me that we rushed out of the house so fast that none of us left any explanation as to where we were going. I decided to call Debra to let her know what had happened and to see if she was all right.

"I can't talk right now," she said.

"Okay, that's all right," I said as we hung up. This was typical of Debra, never available for conversation. I was the one who almost died, and I was the one calling to see if someone else was all right. What was wrong with this picture?

I decided to let her be. I went back into myself and my feelings of elation. I was high from my near death experience. I was high from the adrenaline. I wanted to talk to someone, but no one was around.

Mike returned with a clean change of clothes, food and filtered water. It was almost midnight. He stayed a while to get me settled. We talked but I don't remember what about. Maybe about Debra and how she acted when I called her. Maybe about how close it was this time, even though we had numerous occasions before when I felt like I was going to pass out because I could not get enough oxygen.

The nurse came in and told us it was time for Mike to leave. We kissed each other good-night. He left and I lay there in the silence, unable to sleep. I stayed up all night; all I could do was think. I kept replaying the near death experience over and over in my mind.

I heard a man's voice down the hall yelling, "Take me, take me."

I blocked out his distress. I remembered how I felt on the "other side"—a peacefulness I cannot describe because there are no words. I had no more fears. Every negative feeling had been erased, leaving only joy, peace and a sense of no longer being alone. Bliss. I didn't want to leave this peacefulness I was experiencing. I had only been "there" for what seemed like seconds, although the hospital records report it took them thirty minutes to revive me. They had been the most blissful moments in my life. But I had no choice but to come back. My number had not been called. My time on this earth plane was not yet up. I was needed down here for some reason I did not yet understand.

I then remembered my mother throwing me back into my body, and I smiled. Although she had died twenty-seven years earlier, at that moment I realized she had never really left me; and would always be with me.

The so-called mirage I had seen coming off Carolyn's body was all the blocked energy that she kept locked inside. We both knew she needed help, we just didn't know that what she needed was a God-jolt. When you need help, you need help! That is what Carolyn needed in order for her body to be turned around.

I finished packing my house for our move, which was just two days away. Moving is always so emotional and with what Carolyn and I had experienced over the weekend, I was grateful my mother-in-law, Ruby, was coming to help with our move.

Needless to say, I was consumed and overwhelmed with my emotions.

Immediately after my release from the hospital, I left for Toronto to see a psychologist who understood energy fields and how they can affect the body. I decided to take the trip by car with Mike and our friend, Mary Lou. It was night, she was driving, and we passed what I assume was an electric billboard sign flashing YOU CAN HEAL YOURSELF in huge letters. I thought, "Is this message for me?"

"Did you see that sign?" I asked Mary Lou.

"What sign?"

"Big electric letters flashing 'you can heal yourself.'"

"Nope. No sign."

I convinced her to wait and see if it would flash again. After several minutes of watching, it never re-appeared.

Prior to leaving for Toronto, the psychologist had suggested that I bring a lay-out of my house plans. His main concern was to find out what was causing my body to react to something significant in my environment, most probably around my house.

After our first session, he reported that the energy in and around my body was being affected by geopathic stress.

"This is a natural phenomenon that comes from the energy of the earth or the sky," he explained. "Indians would never have put a teepee on your property. Geopathic stress can also occur with the disruption of energy through man-made neighborhoods."

Using kinesiology, he discovered that I had high levels of geopathic stress in the major areas where I was during the day, and the highest level passed right through my side of the bed. No wonder I was so affected at night. I hated to go to bed. I felt strange walking in my bedroom at night, but not in the day. Even when I felt peaceful, there was a very subtle level of disruption. The psychologist explained to me that I needed to bring these geopathic stress levels down to the point that my body no longer felt disrupted so it could heal.

It sounded crazy, but I had nothing to lose. After years of treatment by the traditional medical establishment, my condition had only worsened. It made sense that the trouble was with my house, because I hadn't had my condition until I had moved there. No matter how absurd they sounded, I resolved to try his suggestions. He told us we would need (now, don't roll your eyes) about fifty pounds of quartz crystals, some sheet metal, some copper coils, and he told us how and where in the house to lay these out. After balancing my body with universal energy, he advised me not to go back into the house until these items were laid in the appropriate places; otherwise it would pull my body back out of balance.

Mike was ready to try anything and felt it was best to buy all my new paraphernalia in upstate New York. That way, when we got back to our home in Atlanta he could immediately align these items to correct the imbalances in our house plans. With the last item in place, I was able to enter the house, and from that day forward, was able to begin to heal.

We had suffered illness all our lives-"out of the cradle endlessly aching". As twins, Carolyn and I often got our childhood illnesses together. Measles, mumps, and chicken pox are common to all children; but what set our house apart as a "sick" place was our mother's lupus. She suffered from this autoimmune disease for many years and her fight became our most imprinted memory. Although I know it was not intentional, when my mother didn't feel well, we children became the targets for her silent aches, pains and complaints. The burden of her illness along with trying to raise four young daughters made anything resembling "normalcy" impossible. It was difficult for all of us, including my dad, and illness ruled our home. We all walked around on eggshells.

Luckily I had my twin sister, Carolyn. We were best friends. We told each other everything; that is, except for our fears and angers about living with a dying

mother. Those feelings lay dormant deep inside both of us, until much later.
Sometimes, when I was really scared, I could feel a presence guiding me in my
confusion. Hindsight tells me those were the moments when God chose to walk with
me. At that time I was scared and unresponsive; I didn't know what He wanted.

I have always had a relationship with God, but as a child it was through my
religion. We were raised in Charleston, West Virginia in a Jewish home. One of the
rituals we did within our home was to keep kosher. Our friends thought that was
strange; and that made me feel embarrassed and different. Unconsciously, and very
slowly, I began closing the door on religion. Thus, my separation with God and religion
began. God, on the other hand, was not going to let me off the hook that easily. He
continued showing me He was there, no matter how many doors I slammed in His face.

If I could write my journey backwards, I would be well and have no
journey. But that only happens in fairy tales. Where and how do I begin?

The first image that comes to mind is seeing and living with a mother
who was sick. Then my mind flashes to--did I have an ordinary life up until my
mother got sick? Well, no. It didn't really start out as ordinary, because I started
out not as a "me," but a "we." Through hypnosis, Marilyn and I have sat in
silence and taken our senses back to where it all began, in the womb, and both
of us could feel each other's presence as well as one another's heartbeat.

I think our toddler stage was probably normal enough. Our sister Natalie was fourteen months older, and to this day I feel that she wanted to be an only child. She was the first born and the first grandchild. She really must have gotten a lot of attention until "we" came along. Twins automatically get attention. It's always, "Ooh, look at the twins! Are they identical?" People always stop to ask questions about twins. Anyway, Natalie's stardom fell when we came along.

As Carolyn said, she and I can remember the other one's presence as far back as the womb. I felt like I didn't have enough room, and to this day I need my space. I do not like cramped quarters or stuffy rooms with a lot of disorganization. I like neat, orderly rooms. Even as I write about this, I begin to squirm in my seat and cough a little. I still get a bit "choked up" just remembering my cramped and crowded beginning.

Two days before Carolyn and I arrived, my mother's brother, Ralph, who was a doctor, examined her and said, "You're doing fine, and so is the baby." No mention that the baby was to be babies. From the very beginning we were a surprise. To this day I just love to be surprised.

Carolyn already mentioned that we have an older sister, Natalie, who was none too thrilled to have two more sisters with whom to compete for attention.

Five years later, we were blessed with another sister, Debra. That was the end of procreation for the Levine family, and a year after that, our mother began to get *sick. She always seemed to be cranky and yelling and I felt very unloved. However, I was especially happy that my best friend, Carolyn, was always at my side to help me through those dark moments.*

The best thing about my childhood was my built-in playmate and best friend, Marilyn. We had other friends in the neighborhood but as far back as I can remember, Marilyn and I always had that "special" bond.

People often asked, "What's it like to be a twin?" I don't know; I've always been one.

We dressed alike until fifth grade, and the only way our parents could tell us apart was by the color of our tennis shoes. The trick was to know who wore the red tennis shoes, and who wore the blue. An added twist was that every year we switched colors. (To this day, we still prefer tennis shoes.)

We shared the same bedroom and the same adventures. We shared care-taking duties for all the animals we acquired, from dogs to frogs, ducks, chickens, hamsters, and our next door neighbors' flying squirrels and wild crow, Spookie. We both liked the unusual.

We had our own language. Marilyn would start a sentence and I would finish it, or vice versa. I would say, "Let's go play hop-scotch," and before I could finish the word "go," Marilyn would be out the door with the chalk in her hand.

We were always laughing at each other, with each other.

When I came down with the measles (or was it the chicken pox?), well, it didn't matter because whatever I got so did Marilyn. To top it off, the parents in our neighborhood had their children come be with us so they could catch these childhood diseases quickly and be done with them. At an early age, illness was rewarded. We got to stay home from school because we were sick, plus we had each other so we weren't alone, plus we had other neighborhood visitors.

I don't remember a lot about Mother's illness. All I remember is that she never seemed to be doing well. Our dad had been taking her to different clinics, but she wasn't responding to the treatments and medications. Death was never discussed in our house, but as kids, we knew something was going on; something was definitely wrong. There never seemed to be any laughter. Mother couldn't do anything with us. She couldn't take us to school, she couldn't be outside in the sun watching us play, and she couldn't take us swimming. She seemed to always be angry and irritable. Her whole body looked swollen. Her hands shook when she tried to feed herself. She didn't have patience with me, us, or kind words. She always seemed to be yelling.

It seemed as if I was growing up with a dark, evil secret--my mother was dying.

I knew Mother didn't feel well, but her crankiness only kept me at arm's length. Her illness showed up through mean and unkind actions. I always felt like she was yelling at me. I didn't feel loved. The sicker my mother got, the more distance I put between us.

Dad never discussed Mother's condition with any of us. It was like a secret, like growing up with an alcoholic parent. You want to say what's on your mind, but you don't dare. That secret set a very big pattern in motion for my life. It taught me to hide my emotions, to suppress whatever it was I wanted to say. I didn't want to "make waves" or cause any conflict. I wanted to be a good child so maybe I would get noticed. The truth was, I needed a hug and for someone to tell me I was loved. I needed to hear that everything was going to be all right, but I never did. The pattern of suppressing my needs deepened. I even began hiding them from myself. They just weren't important.

I later found out that our parents didn't talk to us about Mother's lupus or her terminal condition because they didn't talk to each other about it either. That changed one night in October of 1963, when two of Mother's siblings were visiting. Her condition must have taken a severe turn, because around three a.m. I heard her yelling, "Hurry up, hurry up."

I could hear her talking to God. As Marilyn and I lay still in our beds, we knew our mother was dying. It was cold, dark, and we were alone. Although we had each other, we didn't speak at all. I wanted to run to my mother to tell her I was there to help, but I didn't. We just lay frozen in our beds.

Marilyn and I were simply overcome by our emotions. Maybe we were even experiencing our mother's emotional pain and her turmoil of leaving her children behind. I was angry that Mommy was dying, and she was leaving me behind.

"Hurry up, hurry up." She wanted to go. She wanted to be out of her pain. She was ready.

As I lay in bed hearing her last words I felt breathless. My thoughts were, "Go ahead Mommy, leave!"

I angrily thought, "God, take my Mommy. God lift Mommy out of this pain. God take me out of this pain hearing my Mommy die."

I cried and cried. I was afraid. I was fearful and very angry about no longer having a mommy. After a while, it got very quiet and in the silence I knew my mommy was gone. I felt relief. I felt glad. Marilyn and I lay there in the cold, still room until daybreak.

We heard mumbling of voices in the other room. My dad was with our other sisters. They were crying. They came into our room and told us that our mother was no longer with us. I must have had a blank look on my face, because the only words I remember are my older sister's, saying to me, "Don't you have any feelings? Why aren't you crying?"

I remember thinking, "I've only been up all night listening to Mommy's pleas for help and the echoes from her last words." Everyone in the house, including my father, was sleeping through Mommy's experience except Marilyn and I. I wondered how everyone could have slept through her pleas. In an emotional void and feeling the sting from my sister's harsh words, I ran out the door. Everyone was hurting.

The next thing I remember is that we were rushed to our neighbor's home while preparations were made to take my Mommy to the funeral home. I remember looking out of the window and seeing a long, black car in our driveway. I never saw my Mommy again.

The funeral was two days later. I don't remember receiving one hug or hearing that "everything is going to be all right." After the funeral, I rarely heard my mother's name mentioned again.

We were glad that it was over--all the pain and suffering. We already felt different because we were twins and Jewish; not having a mother just added another dimension to our differentness.

I, too, remember that cold night in October of 1963. All the suffering I saw her go through and the smells from her decaying body came to an end. I felt relief.

It was dark outside when I heard my mother's last cries. She was yelling to God to hurry up, hurry up. My body stiffened as tears tried to surface, but they never did. Carolyn and I shared a bedroom, and neither one of us moved. I lay there unable to respond in any way. I remember just holding my breath, unable to consciously take in air until finally I heard footsteps in another part of the house--another sound to break the icy grip of my mother's dying words. Our father came to our room with Debra and Natalie to tell us Mother had died, but I was still and unresponsive. I lay cold and stiff—I already knew.

The rest of that night and the next day is a blur. We were rushed to a neighbor's house so our dad could make the final arrangements for Mother. We never saw her again. Debra, Carolyn and I were not invited to our mother's funeral. Our father consulted with the rabbi and they decided we were too young to attend. (Maybe this was another reason why I pulled myself away from religion.) There were no good-byes, and nothing was ever going to be the same.

When my mother got sick, Carolyn and I were starting the first grade. I didn't grasp basic concepts from an early age. I had trouble with the three "R's": reading, writing and arithmetic. In the first and second grades I failed all three subjects. I still wonder how I ever passed into the next grade; and why no one noticed that I couldn't read or write and was still counting on my fingers.

My painful childhood memories of feeling stupid followed me into adulthood with such problems as keeping my finances in order. However, these hardships I encountered as a child have become the driving force behind my perseverance today. I have turned my hardships into my challenges.

Schooltime was not only painful because of my learning difficulties, but I had become shy and withdrawn. It was as if I experienced two different personalities. With my neighborhood friends, I was strong--a leader. I explored my strengths as the boys and girls played army. We had our own girls' army and I felt powerful as the leader. Within my family unit, though, I felt lost, weak and helpless.

The dynamics of one's personality can get quite confusing. Confusion became a dominant thought process for me. Deep inside me, I ached for the guidance from a kind, loving role model that would never leave me.

When we were five years old, Marilyn and I, along with some other playmates, had a restaurant at a neighbor's house. We served breakfast and lunch; and donated the money we made to a children's organization. We all thought we made the "big time" when we got our pictures and an article about our restaurant project in the local newspaper.

We grew up in a great neighborhood filled with lots of fun and outdoor activities. Cowboys and Indians; "war" with girls' vs boys' armies, bike riding in the woods and sneaking into a cow pasture behind our house to feed the baby calves are just a few of the good memories.

One of our neighbors was Monique. Her family was French and her dog, Duke, only knew commands in French. Duke could even ring the doorbell.

One Saturday, Monique, Marilyn and I had "school" in our basement. We made all the kids in the neighborhood come to our school on Saturday, so we could "teach" them. This was ironic, since I was having learning difficulties in "real" school; nevertheless I still devoted my Saturdays to our neighborhood school. Even then, I enjoyed teaching others, and found a way to express my creativity. I don't remember teaching our "students" anything special other than what we created. There was no protocol.

One special project involved reading and self-regulated learning. We made up our own stories and put them on 5 x 7 cards, color-coded them, and arranged them in graduated-learning difficulty. We put multiple choice questions at the end of each story. I remember one story we made up was about John Glenn, the first astronaut to orbit the earth. I must have been so creative outside of school because "real" school was an absolute nightmare.

Marilyn and I started school at age five. Even though we weren't too successful academically, we were still passed to the next grade. To this day, I am not sure how this came about. I don't remember our parents ever once being called to school to talk about our grades. In fact, I can't recall any attention at all spent dealing with these matters.

In the fourth grade, I had a teacher who I felt really picked on me. I now believe that she was just trying to teach me; but to a little girl this was humiliating and embarrassing. I cried every day when she asked me to come up to her desk. In front of the entire class, she would say, "What's wrong with this sentence?"

I would stare at my handwriting on the page, wondering, "What is wrong with this sentence? What answer does she want from me?"

She would repeat the question over and over and each time my response was the same--tears. My self-esteem was shattered and I carry this scar to this day. It still affects me in many ways. To this day I have trouble being the center of attention in groups. I do not like to read in front of a crowd, or even at a small family gathering. It has caused me to question myself all throughout my life.

"Why can't I learn like other people?"

"Why is it so hard?"

Despite my problems in school, I remember one good thing. As Marilyn and I entered the classroom one day, we noticed another set of twins in the back of the class. We gravitated towards our soon-to-be new friends, Jane and Jan.

We had lots of fun, calling ourselves "The Twinettes"; and even entered talent shows dressed alike. We sang the song "Let's Get Together," from the movie "The Parent Trap." We all continued to be friends throughout grade school and junior high. When they moved away, we continued to visit. Eventually they moved back, and to this day we still see them from time to time.

In fifth grade we also started to attend Hebrew School. It was expected of you if you were Jewish and planned to be confirmed. The best thing about going to Hebrew School was meeting another set of twins, Donnie and Dougie, who we could never tell apart. Of course I had a crush on one of them, but I don't remember which one. Shortly after we met them, they moved away.

The worst thing about Hebrew School was that the writing moved from right to left instead of left to right. It should have been perfect for me since I already saw things "backwards" because of my learning difficulties; instead I only became more confused. I struggled through Hebrew School for the next two years. I didn't do too well. I never understood why we had to be tested on religion, or on our beliefs.

I was failing at two schools; and at home my mother's health was failing, too. Failure was beginning to have an emotional impact on how I perceived my world.

The good that came out of all this early discouragement was, despite my feeling of academic hopelessness in later years, it prompted me to achieve two post-graduate degrees. Thank you, fourth grade teacher. Somewhere deep in my soul I knew I wasn't stupid. It wasn't until I was thirty years old and working on my second post-graduate degree that I discovered I had learning disabilities.

This important discovery came about as a result of my studies in ophthalmology. I noticed that when working with some children's vision, they read words backwards. I took this concern to my teachers, who replied, "This is normal, and they will outgrow it."

I wasn't satisfied with this answer. There was a Learning Disability Department on campus and I made an appointment with the department head. After voicing my concerns and mentioning that I had similar experiences while trying to learn, she told me, "You have learning disabilities. How did you get through a masters program and get enrolled in another post-graduate program?"

I laughed and then began crying. The tears came from all those years of feeling stupid, of beating myself up because I couldn't learn like others, of putting in long hours for tests and barely making passing grades. The tears also expressed my relief. I wasn't masochistic—I really wasn't stupid after all. Now those many years of struggling had a name.

At first I thought the professor meant I had brain damage, but she explained what learning disabilities are. I was also happy when she told me that most people with learning disabilities usually have high IQ's. My heart soared; after all these years, maybe I, too, was smart!

Back in the early '60's, it seemed that most children had two parents. Among my childish perceptions were feelings that divorce wasn't an "in" thing and that our parents were too young to be dying. Mother's death generated a lot of fear in both Carolyn and me; fear that has surfaced time and again throughout our lives. The re-surfacing of this fear is one of the reasons I have decided to come forth with my story. It is my hope that reading this will help you with insights about your own life and how you are living it.

Pain was my teacher. It is still is my teacher. I created pain in my body for twenty-seven years. I applaud myself for doing such a good job. But why did I do that to myself?

First of all, I wasn't aware that I was doing it. Shortly after my mother died in the fall of 1963, I hurt my back in physical education class. It was a real physical injury, and the pain left me immobilized. I didn't break any bones, but what I was set up for were some major challenges to learn from and overcome. Several weeks later, I got my first menstrual period. I was only eleven years old and these three major events all *happened within an eight-week timeframe. The pain from my mother's death, combined with the physical pain from my back injury and the need for emotional support to help me deal with my first period, were all overwhelming.*

For my aching back, my dad found an orthopedist. I was diagnosed with a condition known as scoliosis, curvature of the spine. The treatment of choice at that time was for me to wear a back brace. I was told by the doctor I would have to wear that brace for two-and-a-half years or until I stopped growing. The scoliosis diagnosis and the prospect of the back brace made me a lonely, scared and very shy child who began to retreat inward.

An interesting parallel event took place for Carolyn right around the time I hurt my back. She broke her nose doing the same exercise. Our accidents happened just a few days apart. Was this a coincidence, (what is now recognized as a typical twin occurrence) or was there something more to learn from this? I've heard many times in my life that there are no coincidences, and I now believe that they are just God's way of saying hello.

Carolyn's nose broke not just once, but four times over the next year-and-a-half. (Hello-red flag going up. Pay attention.) This became a message that needed to be interpreted; but for now, our bodies were beginning to accumulate our life's challenges.

So the dance began, our bodies and spirits intertwined. Our traumas became our dramas.

In the fourth grade, our teacher's desk was on a platform. Carolyn sat closer to the front of the room, whereas I sat in the back. It seemed like every day our teacher would call Carolyn to the front of the room and ask something regarding her English homework. Carolyn often used double pronouns; for example, "My father he." Carolyn repeatedly got reprimanded for this.

I felt sorry for her. I could see what the teacher was asking, but felt helpless to assist Carolyn. All Carolyn could do was cry. In retrospect, I think an insightful teacher would have seen a connection between Carolyn's "twinness" and using a double subject, and been able to communicate the problem in Carolyn's own terms. Carolyn and I even called Miami "Ourami" when we were little.

I remember that the other children looked at me as if it were I being drilled by the teacher. I began feeling like it was me, and blushed during Carolyn's pronoun traumas. My face would get so red I thought I would pop. Hindsight tells me this is when the boundaries of who I was at the time began fading. I was no longer a twin, a duplicate, but I was ONE. It seems as if society, the other children, even our own family considered us one. Is it any surprise that my lost identity became one of my challenges in adulthood?

The following year, the school system decided to separate all twins. I remember that day very well. It was sunny outside and I was sitting in my new classroom with my classmates and all I could think about was Carolyn. It was the first time she was not visible to me in the classroom. It was my first recollection of missing her. I wondered what she was doing, whom she was sitting next to and if she was happy. I was not. I felt frightened, sad and alone. My thoughts that whole day were about Carolyn. Looking back, I applaud the school system for separating us. Should we have been separated earlier? Was it really the best choice to separate us? I don't know for sure, all I do know is that it gave me my first experience of feeling independent. For me, it was a very necessary step.

After Mother died, my dad seemed to respond very quickly. Before you knew it, we had a governess. She was a tailored sort of woman; emotionless in facial responses and very stiff in personality. She wore her hair in a French twist and her dresses were very clean and "proper." She seemed "weird" to me, and I don't remember one friendly thing about her. A favorite television show of mine at the time was "The Farmer's Daughter." The program centered on a governess who cared for a widower's children. They ended up falling in love and the rest is history. In my mind's eye, I couldn't let this happen to our family.

Much to my relief, my dad started dating a young, vivacious woman. They got married near the end of 1964. Her name was Roberta. In the eyes of a twelve-year-old, the picture looked perfect. My life seemed to be getting back to normal.

My dad seemed happier too. The only one of us who had problems with the new arrangement was my older sister, Natalie. Roberta and Natalie butted heads. There was constant conflict. My dad was between a rock and a hard place with nowhere to move.

This triangular drama with my dad, new mom and older sister continued for eight years. My big sister was a tough kid to live with, and although my dad always seemed to respond, he couldn't please both his wife and his daughter. Our new mom did the best she could, but she was also in a no-win situation. As the drama wore on, I tried to live my life as if I was somehow detached from it.

As my family members interacted, I always felt like I was sitting on the sidelines. I didn't know how to participate. I still wonder if I was simply shy, or stuck in a back-brace just thinking I couldn't participate, or if I was perhaps living out my deceased mother's role through the vision I kept alive in my memory of her watching from the sidelines. (How much imprinting from your childhood have you brought forward through your senses to be healed?)

I watched my sisters happily gather around each other on rare occasions; laughing, singing and having fun. I never felt a part of those joyous occasions. As I look back, I wonder to myself, "Why did I just sit on the sidelines?" I vaguely remembered all the dancing around, as I silently sat stiff in my backbrace. I was extremely sad that I could not be like my other sisters, joyfully dancing and clowning around. This became yet another challenge for me to overcome. My challenges were piling up.

The funny thing about being a twin is that when one experiences something, the other one experiences it, too. Carolyn and I have a little joke that it was "like the blind leading the blind"; neither of us knew what direction to take. Both of us have always felt as if we were "hatched" and then just let go to find our way. We unconsciously continued to pass our "unstable health conditions" back and forth, thinking it was just because we were twins. That was the two-step dance that Carolyn and I continued until our mid-thirties. That's when God said, "This is enough. These girls need help." At least that's what I think God said.

We moved to another side of town after Dad remarried. I remember the sadness I felt when we moved, having to leave all my familiar friends behind. It was January 1965 and Carolyn and I started a new school in the middle of the year. It was our birthday, and none of our classmates knew to wish us Happy Birthday. To me, birthdays are so important, because it is a special time to celebrate and give thanks for your birth. I was lucky to have Carolyn. We wished each other Happy Birthday and silently mourned, feeling lost and lonely.

Trauma or drama, any way you want to look at it-- that has been the story of our lives. Our duality. Not just mine and Carolyn's, but for all of us.

I didn't know why we were creating trauma and I didn't know how to interpret it. I did wonder why I couldn't be like the other children. Why did I have to be so different? I not only didn't have a mother, but I was wearing a back brace that felt bigger than I. I was a scrawny kid of about sixty-five pounds toting around a "saddle." At least that was my impression of myself. In the eighth grade when I got braces on my teeth, I really felt like a horse, wearing a saddle with a metal bit. (Carolyn always said she wanted a horse; she just didn't expect it to be in human form.) We all are aware of how cruel kids can be when someone is different. As they teased and made fun of me, I retreated even more. Thank God I have allowed myself to feel those painful memories and recognize that those taunts were NOT about the "real" me. However, that has taken several years of unfolding to recognize and heal.

It has been through my struggles and challenges that I have been able to see the purpose of all my pains. With my awakening into consciousness, I saw that Carolyn and I had been wrapped up in each other's illness throughout our lives. Of course, then we didn't know that we were being blessed with opportunities to grow. Only as I look back over my life can I see how perfect God really is. We are born into our families to learn. Life is hard enough, but our real growth comes from the people closest to us. As I was growing up with all the inconsistencies and dysfunction from my own life, I was learning lessons. If anybody had told me that at the time, I would have thought they were nuts; but it's true.

We all have a book inside of us just waiting to be birthed. I say that because I believe we all have something to teach others. None of us knows everything and yet, we all know everything. That sounds like a contradictory statement, but this is a fundamental TRUTH. All of us have the ability to tap into universal consciousness, the one-mind, the one-psyche, the God-head, whatever you choose to call it. All the knowledge is right inside each and every one of us. Unfortunately, that brilliant, magnificent part for most of us lies dormant.

That is another reason why I have decided to write this book with Carolyn. I want to share my ideas, beliefs, knowledge, discoveries and insights with others. We want to share with others how, in the blink of an eye, our whole world changed. It was as if we went from one reality into the depth of wisdom; and at once we knew more about life, people, illness, wellness, and understood the evolution and journey of mankind. I didn't have all the answers; I just had the ability to see how Carolyn and I and all of us are the creators of our life's circumstances. Everywhere I looked, it became clear that I was either the teacher or the student, and either role was fine. I was starved for knowledge, but equally hungry to teach it. I was surrounded by love everywhere. How had I missed all this before?

This new awareness took on another form of movement for me. I felt light,

happy and free-flowing. . .suddenly dancing with life. I felt like an entirely new person.
God had been knocking at my door for many years. I was either not at home or I wasn't
listening. I didn't know what He wanted, so out of ignorance I had chosen to lie still.

I was happy when Daddy married Roberta. She was young, she was alive, she was fun, and she was what I needed. I fell in love with her. I was so hungry for love and attention. I soon found myself enmeshed to some degree in their lives. When they had difficulties, I quickly became the peacemaker, the "patcher-upper," because I didn't want her to leave. When Roberta came into my life, I began to blossom. I began making other friends in school and also began developing my "separate self" from Marilyn.

After our move, Marilyn and I regressed back into our dependency on each other. We missed our friends, our home, and our neighborhood where I felt safe and protected. It was a difficult adjustment for both Marilyn and me. Natalie, on the other hand, seemed to quickly fit right in with the "popular group." She didn't seem to care that her twin sisters felt lost. Why should she care? They had each other, they always did. After all, Natalie had won back the attention she lost so long ago.

Within a couple of months, Marilyn and I started to adjust. We began to make new friends, but never passed an opportunity to go visit the friends we left behind.

In the spring of eighth grade, all students were given the standard tuberculosis x-rays. My test results showed something on my lung, and I was scheduled for exploratory surgery at the end of the school year. Because this was so scary, in Marilyn's own way, she wanted to cheer me up. She decided to give me a surprise party. I remember walking into a room full of my friends and running out and crying and sobbing. I had interpreted this as a "going away party" for me in case I didn't survive the surgery. I was devastated! How could Marilyn do this to me! My father found me outside and took me for some ice cream. This gesture continued to be part of our private ritual throughout my high school days. I ended up going back to the party and having a great time. One of my friends, Nancy, had a picture taken of a guy I had a secret crush on and she had it blown up to an 8 x 10 as a gift for me. I was so excited to get this present!

I checked into the hospital two days later for my surgery. It went well. One of the doctor's orders was that I was not to see any family members for the first three days after surgery because he wanted me quiet. To a thirteen-year-old who had lost her mother fourteen months before, who had been afraid that she wasn't even going to live, that rule seemed quite unnecessary and scary; since on top of everything I woke up with a paralyzed left arm.

Maybe that's why to this day I find it difficult to follow rules. I feel rules don't have to be so rigid and that people who make them can bend them. At least the nurses let me sneak a phone call to my family on the second day post-op, and soon afterwards I was able to have visitors.

The doctor told me I would not be discharged from the hospital until I could better move my arm. Someone came to my room twice a day to help me raise it up and down several times. That was the extent of rehabilitation therapy in the early 60's. One day while lying in my bed, I got the idea to throw my arm on the wall and let my fingers pull it on up the wall. My self-taught physical therapy continued through the summer, and by fall my arm seemed to be pretty much back in "full swing."

Why is hindsight always so "20/20"? In retrospect, I can see that there were numerous clues as to how my path, my journey, was being molded. There is a metaphysical theory that during the first twelve years of life, you are being exposed to life's lessons; that is, the issues that you agree to work on healing in this lifetime. I'm not sure if I totally agree with this concept. I do believe, however, that hindsight plays a very important role in our learning. As you heal, you are gifted with 20/20 vision to see how your life, your journey, has been playing and unfolding.

My real wake-up call came at age thirty-six. There were other events that could have been instrumental in "waking" me up; but, like most of us, they passed and I got my life back to what seemed normal until the next big crisis appeared. I later learned that crises are only spurts of growth in our consciousness.

What exactly was it that happened to me at age thirty-six that finally got my attention? It was time for me to consciously heal the deep wounds inside my soul. I had already been collecting data by working on myself through therapy. I went into my past pains of growing up with a sick mother, leaving four little girls to a young man who desperately needed someone else to step in and care for them. For some reason, I felt personally responsible for my family. Why I took on that role was beyond my comprehension. In truth, I was overwhelmed with emotions. Nevertheless, this was all in the Divine Plan. Remember that this is now coming out of hindsight.

One of the things I worked on in therapy was my own fear of dying young like my mother. It's always amazes me how early situations can make such a profound impact on one's life. I discovered in therapy that this was all normal, but I still had to deal with my feelings. Feelings that "talk" therapy could not help me move through. It was becoming evident that these emotions were definitely stuck deep in my psyche. I had to ask myself if grieving had become an emotional habit. And, if so, "I" was the only one who could change it. My fear of dying young affected me so deeply that it ricocheted into other aspects of my life. Fear kept me from making commitments in relationships because I didn't want to leave someone like my mother had left my father. At work, fear prevented me from doing a "great" job, so I just did a "good" job, so I would not be so missed if I left.

I also had trouble with change. Fear of change brought up insecurities about starting over, wondering whether I could do it. I especially felt insecure in graduate school when I began new classes. Part of the fear was my learning disability and getting familiar with new teaching methods, but the fear underneath had to do with change and all my insecurities associated with it; including my fears of the unknown.

In therapy and in our own introspection, we slowly take off our veils and masks, to discover what is behind them. I had taken off some of my masks and even thought I had finished my grieving process about my mother's death while in therapy. However, at age thirty-six, I discovered another level of grief that needed to be healed; one that was not described in textbooks. (Whew! Thirty-six was a "big" healing year for me.)

The **Celestine Prophecy**, by James Redfield, says that there are no coincidences, and that behind every coincidence, there is a message. All of these messages add to the pieces of our puzzles, our individual life's journey. We spend our entire life on this pilgrimage. Throughout our journey, we go through peaks and valleys. Learning to work with these "coincidences" can make life very exciting. It can even make our challenges and struggles easier to understand as we piece them together and apply them in our lives. Behind each puzzle piece is a carefully orchestrated part of the Divine Plan.

I finally made the decision to work with God, my Higher Power, and the Universe, instead of against it. In other words, I became aware that I needed to open up my communication with God. I needed to learn to ask Him for help. As I strove towards understanding my truths, I began to notice the valleys more and how they are truly synchronized with my soul's growth.

The night my mother died was a major milestone in my life. Even though some part of me was glad she was gone, her death was a major living nightmare in my life for the next thirty plus years. Looking back with that 20/20 vision, I was glad Mom was out of pain. I was glad for me, too, yet, I so desperately wanted to have a mother. As was typical of all daughters, though, I wanted my mom to be different. I didn't know exactly how I wanted her to be; I just knew that she could not be the mother I needed her to be.

So for me, my second mom, Roberta, was the perfect substitute mom. She made me feel very special and I loved her dearly. With their divorce eight years later, bringing the loss of my second mother, my emotional wounds were "doubling" up. I felt very alone.

As I look back over the years spent with Roberta in the house, I am thankful to have had such an influential role model. From the time I was twelve years old until I was almost twenty-one, I felt like I belonged to a somewhat stable home. I felt loved. I shudder at the thought of how much I could have withdrawn into myself if it had not been for her. I was thankful to her for being there, and even today she plays a role in my life.

The dynamics of our family, with all the hardships that went with it, finally took its toll. My dad and Roberta split up as I was preparing for my third year of college. The split from my parents and losing a mom who I thought loved me hurt me deeply. Like always, though, I seemed to push my emotions deep down where I couldn't feel them. In retrospect, I had done the same thing when my mother died. I truly felt I was not hurt or affected by these women leaving me.

Hindsight tells me differently. Motherloss had influenced my decision on having children. I never thought I was equipped to "be" a good mother. I also thought from a visual point of view, that mothers just leave. The role model I had been playing in my head was definitely not the "June Cleaver" one. Luckily, through maturity, I have enabled myself to heal these past pictures I kept playing in my head. I had to recognize my truths. My mother didn't leave me; she died. Roberta didn't leave me; she and my father divorced. End of story. I have taken the responsibility to heal my past pains and forgiven Roberta and her part in abandoning me. I had forgotten how strong the power of love really is. She had allowed herself to "become" my substitute mother for how ever long (or short) that duration was. Forgiveness was the gift I gave myself to heal my pain over motherloss.

I was an impressionable young lady at the time, and with the split of my parents, I saw that my step-mom had to "start over." She had to find a way to earn a living. I saw that I had been drifting through college and not taking my education seriously. It suddenly dawned on me I had better do something about this. I decided to acquire a skill that would serve me even if I did get married one day. I was accepted into the dental hygiene program at East Tennessee State University for the fall semester of 1972. I had considered studying dental hygiene when I was in high school, but the thought of taking chemistry didn't agree with me. Here I was, three years later, following through with an intuitive hunch I had back in high school.

Shortly after I started the program, my dad married for the third time. My home life dramatically changed. I no longer felt like it was my home, and sadly enough, it was not. Carolyn had been living there while I was at E.T.S.U., and had a lot of conflict with wife number three. It seems, at least in our case, that there's always someone who has to be a thorn in our sides. Carolyn called me, usually when I was studying for a test, to tell me about her family woes. My test scores suffered as a result. I found myself unable to detach emotionally from our conversations. I began to take my frustrations out on Carolyn. I was stern and asked her to stop calling and upsetting me with her problems. I felt guilty, but I knew if I was going to be serious about an education, I had to stay focused. Nothing was going to get in my way. I felt selfish but knew, this time, being selfish was a good thing. It was one of the hardest things I ever had to do!

I graduated in the winter of 1974. I was happy to have my formal education behind me. I was still adrift and not really sure about where to go next. I did know I didn't want to go back to West Virginia. I stayed in Tennessee, and settled for a job in public health, traveling as a dental hygienist among various health departments. That lasted for six months. I knew I couldn't live in a small town in middle Tennessee where even a toothbrush was hard to push!

I packed up my car and headed back home to West Virginia, not wanting to, but not knowing where else to go. I passed through Lexington, Kentucky and thought to myself, "Hmmm! I could live here."

After arriving home, I got my resume together and began sending it out to dentists in Lexington. After getting no responses, I got in my car and drove three hours to Lexington to find a job. Jobs were scarce because Lexington is a college town and *everyone tried to stay there after graduation. I spent a few days looking for a job and learned that a dentist in a nearby town might be hiring. I called him and he said, "How about coming in next week for an interview?"*

I boldly blurted out, "How about right now?" I ended up working for him for over five years.

In 1969, Marilyn and I had both been accepted at the University of Tennessee in Knoxville. It was a big college with over 30,000 students. Somehow, out of all those people, Marilyn and I wound up not being roommates, but next-door neighbors. I felt this was a good thing, because we needed the security of having each other there. However, this security did not seem to help me, and by the end of the quarter I decided to quit college and return home to West Virginia. I wasn't aware of it at the time, but going off to a big college away from home was beginning to awaken my feelings of being alone and lost.

I began to question what life was all about, why I was here, what my purpose was. I didn't know it consciously, but somewhere in my psyche, I knew that Daddy and Roberta were having problems in their marriage. Around that time I started feeling alone and abandoned. By the end of my junior year in college, they had begun divorce proceedings; and by that fall I was overtly depressed.

My happiness from having a great "mother-replacement" had turned into an acute depression. In retrospect, I realize that Roberta coming into my life so soon after my mother's death only masked my feelings and delayed my grieving process. Now suddenly she was gone, too, and that only worsened the inevitable.

I was twenty-one and decided I needed professional help, so I began seeing a psychiatrist. Back then, it was taboo to go to one, as they weren't quite yet understood by society. People just didn't talk about their feelings, and I was bursting at the seams with them. I even went so far as to fly to Pittsburgh each week to see my psychiatrist. That was an hour and a half flight, but I didn't want people to find out I was seeing a "shrink."

Secrets. They continued to follow me. I should have known this was a clue but my 20/20 vision had not yet been developed.

Through therapy, I discovered that I had suppressed my grief over the loss of my mother. Underneath my grief was guilt; guilt for not being able to help her, guilt for wanting her to die, guilt for being glad that she did die, and guilt for me living on. Through all my despair and "survivor's guilt" I had stopped living. My "death" did not happen overnight. It took years for me to slowly stop myself from living. I also discussed my fears with my therapist that I, too, would die young, and how I had a death wish underlying all this guilt.

Off and on over the next ten years I continued with therapy, but it didn't move me past the old familiar pain of losing my mother. Despite my depression, I was able to finish college.

By this time my dad had met and married his third wife, Thelma. I was against this marriage. I was twenty-one and had all the answers. I had begun my grieving for mother-loss (and that included Roberta). I wanted my father to grieve, too. I now realize it was pretentious of me to make decisions for my father, who had his own life and his own decisions. Behind this was my pain and grief. I was hurting badly and I wanted company, or at least someone who would understand.

As the years in Lexington went by, my back pain began to exacerbate. It seemed like every year around the same time, I would become incapacitated in bed for a two-week period. My orthopedist put me in home traction to help alleviate my pain; it eventually passed and I would return to work. I never thought that my physical pain had an emotional counterpart.

After three years of this cycle, I began to question if my hometown orthopedist had been right. Shortly before entering the dental hygiene program, he had expressed his concern about me standing and leaning on a daily basis in order to perform my duties. It was 1978, and a little light went on in my head. I was determined to find my answers.

The personal relationships that corresponded to this time in my life were devastating. I was involved in a serious relationship that I ended after finding out that my boyfriend and a very close girlfriend had been seeing each other behind my back. I was heartbroken.

After that break-up, it was many months before I would entertain the thought of going out with someone else, let alone getting involved. In retrospect, I can see that many times after my relationships ended, I took some time to heal myself. From an even greater perspective, I learned from my dad not to jump back into a new relationship too fast. I learned it is a gift to take the necessary time to get reacquainted with yourself, so in the next relationship you bring your BEST. At that time I didn't realize that I was doing just this, I only noticed the length of time between relationships.

I was in my mid-twenties and most of my girlfriends from high school were getting married. The girls in my office were also getting married and starting families. I often wondered if I would ever meet "Mr. Right." I began to question myself. What was my physical pain trying to tell me? What was my part in all this pain I was carrying? I wanted to know more. Did "it" have an emotional counterpart? (Like my emotions were separate from me.) Was I hiding from someone or something? Was it possible that I was putting out a signal for others to stay away from me? Was I using my pain for protection? During this time, my back pain once again exacerbated, so part of me was thankful that I wasn't in a relationship where I needed to pretend that I felt fine. I found I hid my pains pretty well, including from myself.

In 1978 I got brave and decided to do something else about all the pain I was experiencing by trying another type of doctor. All my life I was taught to see the "right kind" of doctor, that is, the ones who are "approved of" by the medical establishment and society. However, I was desperate. I didn't know who to confide in or even talk to about my decision. I had heard about chiropractors, but I didn't know anyone who went to one. I casually mentioned to my dad that I was thinking about seeing a chiropractor. He told me that I was nuts to even consider it, and said that I could make my "condition" worse or even become paralyzed.

I laugh at that statement now. We have come so far in utilizing different modalities with alternative medicines. It was the 70's and my soul was yearning to be set free. I was beginning a new journey to becoming whole and well. I wanted more from my life and I felt I wasn't able to get it with the way my body was functioning. I felt I had this internal hand picking up the phone, ready to dial. With my father's opinion pushed aside, I took a deep breath and began looking through the yellow pages. I came across a chiropractor with Saturday hours to suit my schedule. I was so scared to make the appointment, but I had to try something new. The old way no longer worked for me.

After my first appointment, I felt remarkably different. I remember thinking I was moving in the right direction. After several visits, I finally felt like there was hope for me; that this person was the answer to my problems. The problem I developed from *that was I began thinking he was the ONLY person who could help me. I gave him my power, no different than with the orthopedist. I was once again giving my power to someone else. It never even occurred to me that I had any power of my own.*

This was my mindset at the time. I didn't realize this behavior was part of who I had become until I moved away in 1981, several years later. I believed so much in a "traditional" way. I believed someone else needed to help me. I believed doctors had all the answers. Emotionally, I felt helpless. My beliefs became like an embedded behavior that took me nowhere. Never once did I question how "I" could help myself. What did I need to do differently? I just lay in my own darkness inching my way to better health.

My experiences in therapy led me to seek out a Master's Degree in counseling. I was determined to help others, to let people know they didn't have to go it alone, that someone did understand.

After completing the Master's program in counseling at East Tennessee State University, (yes, I ended up at the same school Marilyn had attended—we are twins, remember), I began working in Nashville as a social worker at the state hospital's mental institution. I stayed in this job for about four years.

During this time I found a wonderful psychiatrist who helped me move through and finally let go of my depression. Dr. Dave was so special, and he gave me what no other person had before. He provided unconditional acceptance with no judgments. He listened and reassured me that he wasn't going to leave, despite my efforts to push him away. Through his supervision, I began to empower myself. Through self-awareness, I knew I was ready to let go of depression. And I did.

My next challenge was to figure out what to do with myself now that I wasn't going to spend all my time being depressed. Sometimes, as I look back, I think I stayed in my social worker position just to remind myself that I was not really that bad off; that other people had it a lot worse. In some way this work gave me strength. I felt needed, which I didn't fully understand until years later. But it was time to move on, and I searched for a new career.

Everyone I ran into—whether at an airport, at a party, or a new face at someone's house—I asked what they did for a living and how they got there. I didn't want to go back to school if it wasn't necessary. I wanted a more specialized job; something that didn't require me to work nights and weekends, and something I could always fall back on.

One day I was at my ophthalmologist's office and we were talking about career changes.

"Doc, what pays well in this field?"

He told me about the orthoptic/ophthalmic technology program at Emory University in Atlanta.

"Could you write that down?" I asked. "I can't even pronounce those words and my eyes are dilated."

Within a week I had arranged an interview for the program at Emory. I was accepted, and I got frightened. All my old fears resurfaced. What if I died young? Did I want to spend some of my few precious years studying in school? I turned down the acceptance and decided to go back into therapy. This time I tried a group setting, hoping I would not be able to hide my feelings in front of others. I simultaneously scheduled an appointment with a doctor to see if my blood work was normal, and to give me more peace of mind. It was 1980, and I was diagnosed with a positive ANA for lupus. My first feeling was shock and then it rolled into elation and relief. I felt free like a burden had been lifted from me. My mother had died from complications associated with lupus. The big paradox to all that I was feeling was that I now could begin to live my life. I began dealing with all these feelings in my support group sessions with my new friends.

About a year later, I felt emotionally stronger and reapplied to the Emory program. Again, I was accepted, but this time I didn't panic.

I began in August of 1981.

Carolyn and I had been living apart for twelve years when she called to tell me she was moving to Atlanta and going back to school to get another post-graduate degree.

She asked me if I would move and become her roommate. It was the perfect time for me to make the transition because a lot of the people I had been hanging out with had decided to relocate. Lexington had become my home. I had purchased my first house a year before and had become quite comfortable, or at least comfortable with my discomforts.

I had just changed jobs, working with two doctors in two different offices. I thought that would help break up my mundane routines. I also thought that the job switch would help alleviate my back pain. I mistakenly thought that some of the pain was occurring because of the office dynamics in my previous job of five years; but I quickly realized this was not the answer. I began to recognize that my back pain was not the other job but ME. The pain appeared in my physical body; but for some reason, in spite of my having a severe injury, I knew there was more. I was determined to get to the root of my pain.

I truly did not feel my mother's death had affected me the same way it had Carolyn. I was happy that she was happier. Funny, despite my close relationship with Carolyn, I never once gave any thought to how her situation might be affecting me. We had always had parallel situations--like the time we were both rushed to the hospital for the same thing, at the same time- only we were in two different states. It turned out, we both had come down with a terrible case of the flu, sick enough to send us to the hospital. As always, we thought it was "just a coincidence."

I moved to Atlanta with Carolyn in late summer of 1981. I was going to give Carolyn just one year. I rented my place in Lexington to a tenant thinking I would return. I wasn't completely ready to let go. It's amazing how all the events that needed to happen were in sync. (My angels were definitely working overtime with me.)

Within a few weeks of arriving in Atlanta, I found a job working with a dentist, and for the first time in my career I felt like I was in the right place. The dentist seemed a little on the odd side. Odd in the sense, he would come into an examination room to check the patient and he would go right to the problem area before I could utter a word. I often found myself staring at him in amazement. In retrospect I believe he was my introduction to not only listening to your intuition, but also believing in it and following it.

He also had a flip side to his personality that seemed to push all my buttons. I often viewed my "working family" as an extension of my real family. The office dynamic was a great mirror to me, bringing familiar wounds to the surface in order to be healed. All of the stored up emotions that I had physically been feeling somehow got expressed to him. I worked with him for a little over three years. During those years I learned a lot through our "unusual" conversations. For instance, he was the one who told me that I was creating all the pains in my body. Of course I thought he was nuts, really nuts. Who was he to tell me that I was creating my own pain? He didn't know my history of problems, or me. (Sounds like I had ownership over my pain--like I was proud of it, eh?) All he knew was me as an employee. I didn't draw any correlation to my back pain and all my stored up feelings and emotions for many more years, but he was my first introduction into the psychic phenomenon of how the mind and body are related.

In the meantime, Carolyn and I were getting a crash course on coming together to heal as one. We had not shared a living space in twelve years. Shortly after moving in with her, I began questioning if I had made the right decision. We had originally parted from each other to discover who we were as individuals; had we now come together to undo it?

We began fighting, trying to find our archetypal place in our family unit again. I can still vividly see some of the fights we got ourselves into (Sibling squabbles, need I say more?). I can honestly look back and laugh. If God was watching us, (which I know He was) we definitely were putting on a good show. I, personally, didn't want to lose "me;" and I think Carolyn felt the same way. She soon became immersed in her studies and I had a separate life as a working woman. We found our roles once again.

Marilyn and I had been living apart in different states for more years than I would like to count. I felt she was stagnant in her life so I asked her to join me in Atlanta as my roommate. With some reluctance, she said yes.

This was a new journey for both of us. It was scary to come together after all these years of living apart. I feared we would become dependent on each other. Deep in my heart I began questioning myself: "What did I get myself into?" Hindsight tells me it was time for us to come together to heal our wounds. However, this was not revealed to us for another eight to nine years.

There was another reason that I wanted Marilyn near me that I had not shared with her. I had been careful through the years to keep it a secret. Now that we were living together, I was scared that if I told her my secret, she would think I wasn't of sound mind. My secret was that our mother visited me.

As we adjusted to living with each other, I realized that I could continue to keep my secret, as I wasn't yet ready to share it. Other issues began to appear. We began noticing we had similar health issues. We had known that we got our childhood illnesses together, but we found out that even while we lived in different states we continued to experience each other's pains. Marilyn told me about an incident over Christmas holiday. She remembered going home with a boyfriend to visit his family. Prior to his picking her up, she felt she was coming down with the flu. She said she felt really bad, and by the time they reached his parent's home she was very sick. She started vomiting and had diarrhea. This went on for several hours. She ended up in the hospital because of dehydration.

After the weekend was over, she called home and my father told Marilyn that I had experienced those precise symptoms and had to be taken to the hospital at the same time—but I was in West Virginia and Marilyn had been in Kentucky.

Marilyn also said that when she first moved to Kentucky her nose and ears were so stopped up that at one point she was addicted to nose spray. When we moved in together, her allergies cleared up and she no longer needed her allergy shots.

As for me, my nose and ears got all stuffy and I had to seek out an allergist that treated Atlanta pollens. Her allergies had rubbed off on me. We both shrugged our shoulders and thought it was just one of those twin-things.

Our periods came at the same time. This is not uncommon for women living or working together. When we experienced premenstrual syndrome, we went crazy together, neither of us could think, and we were both disoriented and lethargic, among other symptoms. One of my friends in the gynecological residency program suggested that if treated, we both should be treated in the same manner. We thought he was a little "nutty" in his approach, although his insight provided to be one of the first clues for us to look at **the whole picture**. We needed to look at the two of us, together, but we quickly ignored this clue at the time.

The health issues I had been experiencing in Kentucky had changed. I had developed severe allergy problems in Lexington, but suddenly in Atlanta I no longer needed my shots. That was the first of many hands-on courses in life that I would begin to study with Carolyn. This was the beginning of a journey on which she and I were about to embark together.

I lived with Carolyn for three years and never moved back to Lexington. Luckily, I met my husband while working in that strange dental office. I kept hearing everyone else's love stories about how they met their husbands, and now I have a love story too. It begins with a list of all the qualities I wanted in the perfect man—not some imaginary list, but a real, actual list that I kept on a sheet of paper in my wallet.

It was January 1983, my/our birthday, and I was celebrating it with Carolyn at my great aunt's in Florida. It was raining that night. After dining out, I was driving back to my aunt's. I never liked driving in Miami, but for some reason I wanted to drive that night. I let Carolyn and my aunt out in front of the condominium while I parked the car. I was running back to the apartment in the pouring rain, absolutely drenched. I was laughing. I don't remember ever being so wet and having so much fun. Suddenly, I was on the ground and I looked up at a man who had my purse. He must have pushed me down, but I don't remember feeling it. (If you have ever had a car wreck, it was like that with everything happening to me in slow motion. You view the event as happening to someone else. Somehow your body detaches itself from reality.

That was definitely an odd experience.) My immediate reaction was to get my purse back, so I got up and ran after him, to no avail. I was grateful I wasn't hurt very bad, other than having a lot of sore muscles and bruises. Nevertheless, that didn't cover my feelings of being violated. Carolyn woke up the next morning stiff on the same side of her body as to where I had been thrown down. We laughed about it, thinking it was just a twin-thing. The next day, I had to go to AAA to recover my traveler's checks. This was one time my twin identity didn't do me any good. My driver's license had been stolen, and when I was asked for identification I pointed to Carolyn. What good is it when you can't use your own face as identification?

A few weeks went by and I got a call that my wallet had been found. It was mailed to me with all my credit cards intact--everything but my cash and my list. Four months later, I met Terry, my soon to-be-husband. His type had not been on my list, and if I still had it, he never would have had a chance. Again, I smile knowing my angels were hard at work.

I had been cleaning the teeth of a man who reminded me of Captain Stubing on the "Love Boat" television program. I asked my captain if he knew any nice guys to whom he could introduce me. I even mentioned a nice Jewish guy. I have never asked anyone to "fix me up." To my surprise, he said "yes," and a few weeks later I met Terry. My captain arranged for us to meet after they played racquetball at a club to which we both belonged.

I can remember exactly what I was wearing that night- a navy blue tee shirt and baggy sweats. (Not a very sexy approach to meeting a man, but definitely a comfortable one.) I was walking down the corridor when I ran into a female patient from the office. We began walking en route to "meet my man." I had this funny feeling in my stomach and wondered what I was doing, because this woman I was walking with was a knockout. She had all the right curves in all the right places, and a beautiful face to match. Was I crazy? Ehhh…it was too late. My captain had already spotted us coming through the door. I saw the two men in the distance looking our way. Funny, how their tongues were hanging out (a dental hygienist would notice that). I knew they were drooling… and it was not over me. Introductions were made; the captain talked to the other woman, and I talked with Terry.

Our friends left, and we talked for two hours. He asked me out for a date. I said yes, and felt elated as I drove home. I couldn't wait to tell Carolyn about him.

When Terry tells this story, he claims he couldn't wait to ditch the captain and me so he could talk to the other woman. He couldn't believe her beauty. (Just like a typical guy?!) He really wanted to chat with her, instead of me, but he never got the chance. Now we both laugh about our incredible meeting and the little flower placed between us. We became engaged seven months later, and have been together for sixteen years. ***An insight I want to share with you is that sometimes we need to let go of how *we see our lives working out, and just turn it over to a higher power. I did this by placing myself in the position of having my wallet stolen, except that my participation in this was at the unconscious level. So…if things keep "happening" to you, **pay attention**.****

At our wedding, Carolyn gave a wonderful speech, gladly handing me over to Terry. She said, "Marilyn and I started off as wombmates, separated for a while and reunited as roommates. It feels as if I have been carrying her for the first thirty-two years of our lives, and it is time to release her to someone else. Terry, you can take her the rest of the way in!" Her speech had everyone in tears.

Terry became my rock. I had never experienced such a stable person. All I had known was instability.

This is not to say that Carolyn was unstable. She was my first true partner in life. My new partner was not only a different gender, but the dynamics of the entire situation were different. Terry was the first man in whom I had ever confided, and I told him about all the pain I was carrying. He took the whole package, including Carolyn. I feel he was the first man in my life to ever really accept Carolyn, too. I felt very comforted and very loved.

A few months after Terry and I were married, the pain in my body increased. I still had not drawn a correlation about my pain and my mother's death—but my pain usually exacerbated around her death anniversary. My chiropractor suggested that I should consider cutting back on my work. I tried working only three days instead of five, but the pain was not alleviated. My boss and I had not been seeing eye-to-eye for several months, and the emotional turmoil and frustrations had taken a toll on my physical health. I abruptly quit my job. It was December 1984.

When I finished my twenty-seven month training at Emory in orthoptics/ophthalmic technology, Marilyn had already met her soon-to-be husband, Terry. I liked him. He didn't talk much, but he was good to my sister. He was also the first boyfriend she ever had who accepted me. He won our hearts. Right before the wedding, on what was to be Marilyn's and my last night together as roommates, I accepted a date. Marilyn was a little upset that I would go out on our last night together. I said I would be home early. Terry was over at our apartment. The two of them were watching TV, and all of a sudden they heard a loud bang! They both got up and searched the apartment, but could not find from where the bang came. I returned from my date and they told me what happened. They were caught up in telling me the story, and all I could do was sit there and smile—my secret was about to be revealed. Mother had decided to take matters into her own, shall I say, hands. So, nonchalantly I said, "It was Mother."

"WHAT?"

"Yeh, remember I told you she's been coming around for years. I told you briefly and jokingly about her visits when we first moved in together."

All the while, I had this grin on my face. They wanted to know more about what I meant.

I explained to them, "It all started years after she died. I was going through therapy at the time. It seemed she would always show up when I was extremely depressed. I would be lying in my bed, crying, and a PRESENCE would come into the room. What felt like her arms would go around me, and she would rock me. It would only last a few seconds. This presence always scared me. I always knew it was Mother, but I didn't know what she wanted, and I sure didn't know how to talk to her. This went on for years."

The three of us calmed ourselves down. Terry kissed Marilyn goodnight and he left for home. Marilyn and I got ready for bed. She was in her bedroom and went over to close the window shade. As she reached for it, she realized it wasn't there. She looked around the room and found it on the floor, clear across the room. She called for me. I walked in the room and saw what had happened and said, "Ehhh…Mother."

So we did get to be with each other on our last night together in this part of our lives. Mother made sure of it. Because it was so late and Marilyn was moving out the next day, we ended up sleeping together in my bed. WOW!

Mother really has always been there when we needed her, even though she wasn't physically present.

The wedding was the following week. It was gorgeous. Marilyn looked radiant, and her husband Terry beamed from ear to ear with his contagious smile. It was a sit-down dinner. People were giving toasts to the newlyweds. Marilyn looked at me and said, "Are you going to give me a toast?"

I had no idea what to say. I didn't like to speak in front of people, and out of all the people there, I was the only one who knew Marilyn the best. Now she was leaving this partnership and creating another. I don't know what I said. I must have gone into an altered state, although I didn't know about altered states at that time. All weekend we had been hearing, "What is Carolyn going to do without Marilyn?"

The next thing I remember was saying to Terry, "I took her the first thirty-two years, you can take her the rest of the way in."

As I was speaking, I was shaking from all the emotions that flooded me. I rambled about our lives together. I was losing my Marilyn. I looked around the room. The audience was in tears.

"For those who have asked about what am I going to do without Marilyn," I threw my hands up into the air and said, "I'm fine." Everyone broke out in laughter.

After I sat down, people came up to tell me what a wonderful speech I had given. My Aunt Esther said, "I didn't know you could capture a crowd like that."

I had no clue at that time what she meant.

Marilyn moved about twenty minutes away, not too bad if there wasn't a lot of traffic. We saw each other every seven to ten days, but talked on the phone several times each day. She was adjusting to married life, as I was beginning to settle into really being single. I was coming to the tail end of my training at Emory. I had already lined up a job with a local ophthalmologist, and was to begin work the latter part of the fall. When this time came, I started to feel the loneliness, and decided after six months of being single that I should look for a roommate. I never gave one moment's thought as to what was behind my loneliness, and I began to fill the space.

I told friends that I was ready to fill Marilyn's bedroom. This was a big step for me, as I had never shared living quarters with anyone outside my family. I had college roommates, but there isn't much to share in a one-room dorm. I met an attorney, Suzie, from New York, who was looking to move to Atlanta. We decided to give it a go, and she moved in.

Two things stand out about Suzie. She seemed to be on a search for what life was all about, and she ate three healthy meals a day. I thought that was weird.

She didn't eat fast foods, and preferred whole grains and vegetables to processed "junk" foods. Hindsight tells me she showed me what was about to come my way. Five years later I was forced to begin eating healthier. Maybe if I had emulated her eating habits, I wouldn't have gotten so sick, but at that time my blocking mechanisms prevailed.

By the time of Marilyn's wedding, I had met Mike, my husband to be. My roommate, Suzie, decided to move to Israel to continue her search for her true meaning in life. This was another clue that I, too, would soon be delving into a search for my "Self" on a deeper level. But at the time, I was secure with my new career. I knew it wasn't really challenging enough, but it gave me the opportunity to focus on my new relationship with Mike.

Mike was totally opposite from the men to whom I had been attracted in the past. He made me laugh when I got too serious. I told him up front that I would only date him one year, because I was thirty-three and wanted to get married. He was fine with this arrangement. In the past I would have stayed in a relationship way past the healthy limit. This time I was taking charge, or at least that is what I thought.

I also thought our relationship was progressing nicely. We discussed what we each wanted in a spouse. I really thought that he was talking about me when he described his mate—Wrong! We soon broke up.

One of the characteristics that really attracted me to Mike was his ability to process very quickly. He seemed to process problems and come up with logical solutions quickly, on what seemed to me to be any subject. I didn't know if he was very bright, or just very good.

Anyway, we split up and he quickly lined himself up with dates with the type of women he thought he was attracted to. He wanted a woman that was more of an intellectual type. He found, though, in his comparisons with me, that he really liked the strength I showed as we broke up. He called me, wanting to get together, and talked me into seeing him that night. After several "yeses" and then "nos," I reluctantly said yes.

He took me to a Mexican restaurant so I could get my favorite nachos. He told me what had been going on with him in the dating scene, and that he had been out with women who he thought were his type.

As I chomped away on my nachos, he told me he had now realized that he really loved me, and he asked me to marry him. He caught me completely by surprise! It had only been a week since we broke up. (I told you he was quick.) I was very suspicious of what I was hearing and told him I had to think about it. I was really unprepared for all we had been through...me not being the right woman that could meet his intellectual needs, indeed. Two weeks later on Valentine's Day, I said yes.

The week before our wedding, I moved into Mike's condominium. I hated giving up my apartment. I liked the way it overlooked the woods and I felt it was my little house, my safe place. It had been my home for the past five years. That might not mean much to some, but for me that was an accomplishment. Ever since I graduated from high school, I hadn't stayed in one place for more than three or four years, nor had I remained in one profession that long. I was constantly running from myself, always thinking it was going to get better just around the bend. For me to give up my security blanket, my apartment, was something major.

I wasn't very good at going to other people's weddings. It wasn't very different for me this time, except that this was my wedding and I had to be more involved.

The wedding plans became overwhelming to me. I couldn't handle all the conflicts involved in trying to please the different family members. The planning included what food to order for the guests, the dresses, the hair, the flower arrangements and all the rest of the little details. I was ready to explode! As I look back on this period in my life, with my special day approaching, I wonder why I never asked what was underneath all my feelings of being overwhelmed.

I can see clearly now how I missed my mom on this very special day of mine, and I wanted her here with me. I just didn't want to participate. The little girl inside me was pouting and running away.

While the little girl in me pouted, Mike stepped in and made the final arrangements. The night before the wedding I was a basket case. Whatever Mike said to try and calm me down, I responded to with some flippant remark. I did not want to go down that aisle, but I shrugged it off as "bride's jitters." I had a drink (which I don't often do) at our rehearsal dinner and remember thinking, "I needed that!" The rest of the night went pretty smoothly. The next day I overcame my fears. As I began to walk down the aisle with my dad, he softly said to me, "Your mother would be proud of you." Tears welled up in my eyes. For the moment my heart was happy.

As I continued to walk down the aisle, I also knew on some level that tremendous changes were about to unfold. These changes, one year later, began presenting themselves. My wake-up call was about to begin.

And so Mike and I began our journey together. One warm evening I came home from work and Mike was on the phone with his mother. I was hot and tired so I decided to go to the pool for a swim. The pool was crowded. I remember thinking that it was never this way at my apartment complex. I felt the fury building inside me. All I had wanted to do was relax and swim some laps. I wanted some peace.

I stormed out of our condominium and said to Mike, "You will find me at my old apartment; I'm going there to swim!"

It was only five minutes away, but I couldn't wait to get there. When I drove up, nobody was in the pool. As I dove into the water, relief came over me. I was peaceful at last.

This was just one of the incidents we had as I adjusted to his place, and to our marriage. There were many more, but I'm sure the scenarios were not much different than the one I just mentioned. At the time, I didn't know about patterns, and about how we repeat them until we get the lessons(s) behind them.

The memory of my orthopedic doctor telling me I had to accept that I was always going to have back problems kept resurfacing. Even though I had been physically injured, I didn't want to buy into what the doctor said. I don't know where I got that inner determination, but I just "knew." I knew that if I could just get my back stronger, through exercise, I would be a lot better for it.

January was a new month and a new year. It was 1985. It was also my birthday month. I was free at last to explore myself without a job to weigh me down. My first plan of action was to find an exercise program that worked for me. I found an aerobics program nearby and began working out.

I was psyched mentally and emotionally. I had a wonderful time exercising, but afterwards I could barely move. It was as if my vertebrae misaligned with exercise. It was my goal to continue to make my muscles stronger. I exercised for many weeks, followed by several visits to my chiropractor. Reluctantly, I realized that this plan of action was not appropriate. I desperately wanted my body to work with me, not against me.

I took up walking. I had to get my body moving. Some days I did great, and then there were the days I didn't do so well. But that was my body's cycle, to which I adjusted. I had accomplished the goal of finding an exercise program. It wasn't what I had planned, but it was one that worked. Months went by and I was feeling better, so I began free-lancing by filling in for other dental hygienists. This way of working kept me quite busy. My lifestyle had adjusted to me. I found a way for my body to work and to exercise.

At the end of 1986, I felt physically stronger; enough to accept a full-time position again. I found a doctor who wanted me to work for him. I was excited by the challenge of working for a new doctor in periodontics. Within a few short months my back pain worsened. It was the worst ever--my pain had hit an all-time high. It never left me for one moment. I slept on the floor at night in an attempt to get some relief. The mere scooting of my chair towards the patients was unbearable. At lunchtime I would go home just to lie on the floor.

Needless to say, I had to make another decision. I left the practice early that summer, determined to get at the root of all my pain. I visited my orthopedist and explained the severe pains I had been experiencing. He sent me to a specialist, who did a bone scan. The words were never spoken but I thought it possible that there might be a tumor. I was elated to find no real physical cause for all my pain, but I was stunned! Now what? Where would I go from here?

Months went by and the pains would come and go with no rhyme or reason, but I remained determined to find my answers.

At the same time I was experiencing the severe pains again, Carolyn and Mike bought a home closer to where we lived and had begun restoring it. Shortly after they moved in, Carolyn began coughing. Everytime I walked into their home, I smelled gas. A few months later, they discovered there was a gas leak and had it repaired. Carolyn's symptoms seemed to get worse as the renovations continued.

She went to an allergist who ran tests and treated her with allergy shots. Instead of getting better, she worsened. It was as if in one month's time her immune system had broken down. Carolyn and I began doctor shopping. We needed some guided answers, so our journey from sinus specialists to pulmonary doctors to rheumatologists began. We took several side visits to the chiropractor from whom Carolyn found no relief.

At one point, one of the doctors mentioned to Carolyn to watch out for the ecologist. Carolyn wondered what an ecologist was. A friend had mentioned to Carolyn that she needed to get in touch with her metaphysical self. Carolyn joked and said she was having a hard enough time with her physical self. Carolyn and I were some pair. Her respiratory problem and my back problem had become the focal points of our lives.

About six months after Mike and I married, "someone" decided it was time to have a family. I say "someone" because now I realize that I constantly gave my power to someone else, anyone else. I didn't want to take responsibility. I didn't want to participate. I was thirty-five and Mike wanted children. Did I? I thought as the time came closer that I would adjust to having a family. Wrong! All my fears resurfaced about having children and then getting sick and leaving them in death. I saw this happen to my mother. I thought this was all behind me; I thought that I had dealt with this in therapy. Mike and I had discussed these concerns prior to our marriage. We had even consulted a rheumatologist who assured me that I was physically fine, despite testing positive for lupus since 1980. Although the lupus wasn't active all the tests indicated a failing immune system. The rheumatologist told me not to worry, that having children would not push me over the edge.

Who was he kidding? And whose edge? This was 1986 and doctors gave little thought or credence to the mind-body connection. Mike saw how this was so upsetting to me, and together we decided to wait on having a family.

By the end of our first year we had purchased our first house. It had four bedrooms, and all pointed to the probability of considering the family "scene" once again. The day we moved into our house, we saw a double rainbow as we drove there. I mentioned to Mike that there was always a pot of gold at the end of the rainbow, as I silently wondered what that double rainbow had in store for us.

We moved in and began to plan our renovations on our twenty-five year old house. We had already put new carpet down and it had made a big difference to the house. We didn't really need to do a whole lot to the house, just some updating.

Mike started a new job. I had been working two days a week in ophthal-mology and sold real estate for the rest of the week. With my schedule, I decided I could handle work from home and simultaneously supervise the renovations.

For the next four months, I had a lot of exposure to the inside of my freshly renovated house. One day my nose kept itching. I had smelled gas, but Mike didn't, so I ignored it. My nose kept itching, and one day I couldn't breathe through one side. I had the gas company check for a leak and, simultaneously, I went to a doctor. A woman came to check for the leak. She found two small holes in our gas line from the kitchen stove and one leak coming from our gas fireplace. She told me that the brain automatically tunes these types of smells out once it has put out its initial warning signals.

The doctor found my nose was swollen and gave me nose spray, which didn't help. He tried lots of different medications, but nothing gave me relief. Months went by and I still couldn't breathe through my nose. I told the doctor that I had taken allergy shots in the past, and they had helped. I was retested and put back on the old routine and within six weeks I developed asthma. My eosinophil count (an allergic response noted in your blood work) was climbing. My nose was still blocked. Over the next six months, I continued to steadily go downhill. I had sinus infections one after the other. By this time I had started to develop a strong cough.

One day while we waited in the reception room for Carolyn to see a new doctor, she began coughing. It wasn't a full-blown episode, but she got out her breathing machine, which she faithfully carried at all times. As she inhaled on the machine, I looked at her, and with such profound clarity said, "You know Carolyn, we are supposed to be learning something from all of this."

She looked at me inquisitively and said, "Yes, but what?"

That was the starting point of a new and deeper journey that we were about to undertake. We were going to become detectives into uncovering the secrets of wellness.

We didn't have a clue as to how we were going to do this, nor who would be there to help.

Carolyn also had other health problems. She had experienced severe endometrial pains for years and was told she needed surgery. She couldn't have the surgery; she had become too sick.

Another doctor found a tumor wrapped around one of her vocal cords that needed removal. We all thought that could be why she was coughing.

After the removal of the tumor, Carolyn's vocal cord was temporarily paralyzed. She barely spoke above a whisper, and a few short weeks later her cough returned. The tumor had not been the cause of her cough. She was also told that additional surgery might be necessary to repair the space left near her vocal cord. For the moment, though, she needed time to heal. Carolyn ended up seeing a sinus specialist, thinking that the drainage in the back of her throat was the cause of her cough. He did yet another surgery on her. The amount of diseased tissue was incredible. It was removed, but it was not the cause of her symptom. Each time Carolyn had surgery, her immune system was further weakened. Antibiotics exacerbated her symptoms, and each time she went into surgery the doctors put her at risk. She became so allergic to everything in the environment that she even reacted to the disinfectants used in surgery, the equipment, and the plastic gloves. And each time she went back to her home her symptoms got worse. I was always on call. Mike was on beeper. Who was going to help us? Where *were we going to go with this?*

So the dance continued. From the dance with my twin sister, to the dance with my husband, and now, suddenly all four partners were stepping on each other's toes. And no one was leading.

I began some research and interviewed doctors who called themselves ecologists or preventive medicine specialists. I thought these doctors were weird. Their treatment included vitamins and minerals that helped detoxify the body and rebuild the immune system. I was very conventional in my thinking and believed in the traditional medical approach, but it had failed me. I was scared. I needed help and didn't know where to go or to whom I could listen or trust.

Within three weeks, the doctor I chose to work with decided I was too "far gone" for him to help me. He referred me to the Environmental Health Clinic in Dallas, Texas, and arranged for me to go. On December 28, 1988, I went to Dallas in a very fragile health condition.

As we landed in Dallas, one of my coughing attacks began. I remembered from my asthma support group that sometimes flying and changing altitudes could induce an asthma attack. My inhaler didn't work. I tried unsuccessfully to wait for my turn to get off the plane. The attendants had all the passengers step aside as they rushed me off the plane. I hooked up my breathing machine (I always carried it in my tote bag) to an electrical outlet. My face was beet red. I was gasping for air. Strangers looked on as I sucked on the apparatus for dear life. A doctor from the plane approached us and said, "You need to get her to the hospital."

"That's what we are trying to do," Mike said. The breathing machine provided some relief and I calmed down. We quickly found our bags, a cab, and were off to the clinic.

I could never have been prepared for what I was about to see and learn, although, looking back, I suppose I did have some preparation. I had worked in a mental institution, which had provided a basic foundation. I was about to learn that I, too, had become very sick. But how did my immune system get so broken down?

We quickly learned that I had environmental sensitivities. I was allergic to my environment and was called a "universal reactor." I was a sitting duck for the gas leak.

I grew up in a city with lots of chemical plants. My diet was bad; I ate fast foods that had little to no nutrients. Added to this was the everyday stress of a new marriage. The gas leak and house renovations had pushed my immune system over the edge.

I was having trouble bouncing back. The doctor's theory was that a more sterile environment would allow my body to detoxify itself from the overload of all the chemicals; from our foods, water and air that we breathe. He didn't know how long I would have to stay at the clinic. The accomodations provided only the bare essentials. My room consisted of a cot, a small nightstand, a clock radio, and an air machine to clean the air. All apartments had a fully equipped kitchen, table, four chairs, and a bench in the living room. TV and telephones were optional and we opted not to have them. There was no carpet or pictures on the walls. All I could hear was my voice echoing off bare walls. All I wanted to do was sleep and I constantly wondered how I let my body get so far "out of whack."

Mike stayed with me for the first couple of days. Then Marilyn stayed with me the following week. Blood tests revealed that my detoxification pathways had shut down. I was tested for things to which I was allergic. This was completely different than the standard allergy testing with which I was familiar. One substance at a time was injected into me to gauge any reaction. This technique is called provocation-neutralization. My immune system was so shattered my skin didn't even swell from the injected substance.

The only way that sensitivity could be measured was through my symptoms. There was a lot of guesswork and this was very hard. My nose was so congested that I could not inhale or exhale. This continued for the next five weeks.

Marilyn and I couldn't believe what we learned. Many of our symptoms over the years had probably been related to chemical sensitivities.

Marilyn realized that her back problems could have been related to the chemicals she inhaled as a dental hygienist. We got some real "eye openers."

I had trouble with my assigned apartment, and had already moved once. The drain from my bathroom tub was too moldy, and even with the door shut and a towel at the bottom of the door, I became wheezy from mold exposure. The doctor recommended that I move to a place about a half-hour from Dallas, which I called the Tidy Bowl.

When Marilyn and I initially drove up, the manager ran out to us yelling, "Stop, stop, you can't come here. I can smell Tide on your clothes."

I whispered to Marilyn, "If I come here, it will break my spirit."

Little did I know what I really meant about how my spirit would break. Two years later I would find out.

The new "Tidy Bowl" place was very secluded. Each person had his or her own trailer, which consisted of one room with porcelain walls, ceiling, and floors, and a porcelain toilet. Everyone cooked and ate in the same mess hall. Showers were in another part of the campus.

I found it was depressing and lifeless. I couldn't bear it. Mold or no mold, and still coughing, I was going back to my luxurious apartment in the city.

After a week, Marilyn returned to Atlanta and used her newfound knowledge to find a preventive medicine doctor for herself. Being my twin, she wanted to prevent herself from falling into any illness. I remained in Dallas for another four weeks. Marilyn also helped Mike locate another place to live, as my house was simply too toxic. The day before I had just about finished my testing, Mike called to say he had found a house that seemed to suit my needs. It had hardwood floors and we thought we could make it work. He took Marilyn to see it. She didn't feel good about his decision, but Mike didn't listen. He had a sick wife coming home and he was desperate. Before I arrived home, Mike had hired a crew to clean this house with safe products. Safe products are made without solvents, chemicals, or fragrances. It took them fourteen hours. Mike tried to move me in. I lasted an hour and a half before the rageful cough appeared. I couldn't be there. We later learned that the owner had treated for fleas—despite his word that he had never used chemicals in his home. Treating for fleas, bugs, etc. is very toxic, especially to an immune system that has difficulty detoxifying.

The only place where my body did okay was at Marilyn's place, but it was just a two-bedroom condominium and too crowded for the four of us.

We decided to switch houses, but kept our spouses. I really didn't do any better at the condo. But looking back on it, I think I just felt safer with Marilyn's belongings around me.

By the end of seven months, Marilyn and Terry wanted their condo back. They wanted their lives back. They wanted to move forward and could no longer live on hold. Marilyn wanted to sell the condo and find a larger home. She was tired of being trapped in my life. She was already trapped in her own life, by being in back pain for over twenty years. She was emotionally ready for something new.

Carolyn and Mike moved into our small condo. I did my best, we all did. I am thankful for such a wonderful husband who didn't make waves and went along with whatever was requested. And Carolyn was also lucky to have Mike.

I spent most of the days at my condo taking care of Carolyn, still searching for a doctor to help her. I went out for daily walks to keep my body active and moving. I still had pain, but my focus was on Carolyn. Carolyn felt my daily walks affected her condition. My being outside, either on walks or in restaurants with my husband and friends, exacerbated her symptoms. (Is this a twin-thing, or was there something more to be learned?)

Those times were hard on both of us. On numerous occasions, Carolyn and I talked about the difficulties of my having a life outside my relationship with her.

Despite our special bond, I was still trying to lead my own, separate life. I was forced into a bad situation, and luckily I never had to choose. Carolyn and Mike decided to give their first house another try.

This coughing cycle continued for three-and-a-half years. Carolyn and I never once questioned whether there was more to life than what we saw. All our lives we had seen or been around someone who was sick. This "comfort zone" had been imprinted from childhood, and we were just doing the same old dance. Different song, same dance—the patterns repeated. Although Carolyn and I each had a separate wake-up call, the dance still needed to be completed. One of us had to lead and I was chosen.

How does one know he or she is having a wake-up call? What is a wake-up call anyway? If anyone had told me something like what was about to happen was a possibility, I would have said they were nuts. When it actually happens, though, there are no doubts; you just know and you don't question anything. There is just a profound knowingness. That was what it was like for Carolyn and me.

Mike returned to our first house and started to "un"-renovate it. He ripped out the carpet in one bedroom to see if I could even sleep at our toxic house. It worked. As beautiful as the carpet was, we had the installers remove it all.

I was so upset. I didn't like seeing my gorgeous carpet being ripped up. Why couldn't I live with carpet? Why was my body failing me? Luckily we had twenty-five-year-old hardwood floors underneath the carpet. People pay a lot of money for wood floors, and we already had them. I wanted the carpet underneath my feet, though, I didn't like bare floors. I felt naked.

I later learned that this was symbolic. I had to be stripped of everything in order to rebuild. This was the spring of 1989. I was back in my home once again. I was hopeful that I could start to get some normalcy back in my life; whatever that was.

Just because I was back at home did not mean I could sit back and let my body get well. Mike and I had learned a lot at the environmental clinic on how to make our home a safer place to heal. We learned how toxins in the house, the workplace, and our bodies could be causing symptoms.

The clinic staff had also emphasized making our bedroom an "oasis," a place that is totally safe. If the bedroom is toxin free, then the body has a better chance to cleanse itself of accumulated chemicals from the day. Toxins can come in many forms, such as dyes, sprays, petrochemicals, copy machine solvents, perfumes, colognes, etc.

A safe bedroom allowed me to use extra energy to repair damaged organs, tissue, and cells. Another theory behind the "safe" bedroom concept is that this type of environment allows one's body to better tolerate the world's pollution.

We had a lot of work to do to make the house safe. We had already pulled out the carpet, which was full of formaldehyde, glues, and gasses. We went to work on our bedroom. We zipped the mattress into a non-treated cotton encasement and surrounded me with cotton sheets, pillows, and blankets. The furniture was old, so it could stay because all the chemical smells from the materials used to make it had decreased. We added an air machine to remove molds, dust, and chemicals from the air around us. We removed all books and magazines (these have formaldehyde from printing and glues from binding), shoes (these have molds inside them from sweat and chemicals from treated grass), and clothes (these have formaldehyde and solvents from dry-cleaning solutions) from the bedroom.

We then tackled the rest of our house. After we removed all the pine cleaner, bleach, furniture polish and pesticides, we had two large garbage cans filled with toxic chemicals. Included were many items that we take for granted as part of modern day life. It's amazing how many poisons are in our homes and garages. I realized that not everyone had to go to this extreme to get well, but for me, it was what I needed to help my body detoxify itself.

I had already begun to look at my diet at the clinic. At home I stocked my cabinets with whole grain foods such as brown rice, quinoa, millet and buckwheat.

(Remember my old roommate Suzie? This is how she ate and I had thought it was weird.) These foods are not chemically or mechanically processed and have high concentrations of nutrients. Also, I started buying organic beef and chicken. Organic foods have not been treated with any pesticides, herbicides, hormones, antibiotics, or preservatives. I started eating more vegetables, organic ones when possible. As I started to eat a more healthy diet, I noticed my moods became more stable. I had never considered that food was a cause of mood swings. I began drinking filtered water, too.

I learned that eating healthier did not mean I was digesting properly. Sometimes when I ate, I felt a gurgle in my throat. I learned that this indicated either the need for something to help me digest my foods, or that I had eaten too much in one sitting. I was beginning to learn how my body was talking to me.

I settled back into my home with my familiar belongings, and began to consider what I had learned from my fellow patients regarding other healing modalities. Included were methods such as acupuncture, homeopathy, herbs, vitamin and mineral supplementation, oxygen therapies, and on and on. I didn't know where to go or how to begin. I thought if I could get myself aligned, I would and could heal. Because my worst symptom, the cough, was so hard on my musculo-skelton system, I sought out a chiropractor. This is where I began to learn more about how the body operates, and how it is possible for us to access the knowledge that lies within.

I didn't exactly understand what the chiropractor meant when he explained that through kinesiology my body could tell me what it needed to help bring it back into balance. This was a difficult concept for me to accept and understand, but it led me to try other alternative modalities. Over the next two years I tried thirty-three different techniques to assist me back to wellness. They all seemed to work a little bit by making me stronger, but none of them took away the worst symptom—the cough.

During the spring of 1990, I stayed at my parents' condominium in Boca Raton, Florida to minimize my exposure to the heavy Atlanta pollens. I stayed there about two months, and during that time I began yet another series of acupuncture treatments. When Marilyn came to pick me up, I suggested that she try these treatments to see if she could get some relief from the muscle spasms in her back. With much reluctance, she agreed. After her first session, she realized that it did make her feel more relaxed.

Around that same time, I met a woman at the local health food store who did Reiki. This is a laying-on-of-hands healing technique that works with universal energy to bring your body back into balance. When I told her that I had been very sick, she said she thought she could help me. I invited her to the condominium to see what would transpire.

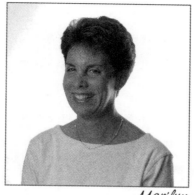

Marilyn

Marilyn's Instantaneous Healing

Wake-Up Call No. 1   Three months earlier

*I*t was May 1990. Carolyn had gone to Florida while Atlanta had its spring-time awakening with its wonderful smells from the blooming flowers and trees. She had been down in Florida for almost two months. I was supposed to pick her up mid-month, but early one Saturday morning I received an urgent call from her. She said that she needed my help because she was scared about the extra adrenaline shots she had been taking. She thought that maybe it was time to return to Atlanta. I flew down the next morning to drive her back. As I got off the plane, I could smell thick pesticides in the air. I wondered if that could be the cause for Carolyn's increased use of adrenaline. I related this observation to Carolyn and she made the necessary adjustment by not spending extra time outdoors.

While Carolyn was in Florida, she had been seeing an acupuncturist. She urged me to give this a try; she was certain it might help alleviate some of my back pains. I hesitated with great resistance because I hated the thought of needles. Deep inside me, however, a little voice questioned, "What if it could help?"

I made the appointment, and Carolyn and I went in together. We had our treatments at the same time but in different rooms. I lay on the table and took a deep breath as the doctor began putting the needles into my body. All I knew about Chinese medicine and acupuncture was that the doctors worked with the "chi" (energy), or life force, by placing needles along the "meridians" of the body. (Meridians, in Chinese medicine, can be understood by imagining the way that arteries carry blood through the body. Meridians carry the "chi" through the body.) Nevertheless, I was scared to death and felt like a dartboard. I was stiff and the needles were painful. I was not yet aware that my resistance made the needles hurt going in. The twenty-minute session seemed like eternity. I wondered if it was working and how I would know if it was, since I didn't feel anything unusual.

I was elated when the doctor came in to remove my needles, and glad to get out of the office. I felt a little more relaxed after the session, but I couldn't tell if it was just the relief from being out of there.

Since we had figured out how to manage Carolyn's health situation a little better, we decided to stay a few extra days so I could get a few more acupuncture treatments. (Oh joy! Can you feel my elation?) I had to be mindful that this could be a really good thing.

After the second acupuncture session, I had planned to meet for a few minutes with Joan, the Reiki healer Carolyn had met. She was going to do an assessment of my energy fields; whatever that meant. Joan and Carolyn thought that might be a good idea, since we were twins. Joan told Carolyn she had never worked with twins before, and that she welcomed the challenge. I thought it would be about a fifteen-minute appointment, so I made a lunch date with a friend. I also thought that I did not play a vital role in Carolyn's health problem or in her overall condition. After all, although we were twins, we were also two people with two very different health issues. Silently, I began questioning the "weird" path Carolyn was beginning to take. I felt I was being pulled in a direction that I had no way of relating to. End of story.

To our amazement, the fifteen-minute assessment turned into a fascinating exploration that lasted three hours. Needless to say, I canceled my lunch engagement.

The session began with Joan seating me in a chair. Carolyn was in the kitchen cleaning up her lunch dishes. Joan put her hands about ten inches away from my body, and moved them around me almost as if she was outlining my body. She told me to breathe nice, even, long, slow breaths, and suggested I close my eyes.

I was in full concentration of my breath when I heard Carolyn start to cough from the other room. My eyes were shut. I kept trying to breathe without losing my concentration. As I continued to breathe, all I could hear was Carolyn's cough getting louder. I began to wonder if she was beginning another one of her attacks. With my eyes still shut, Carolyn popped her head into the room and said, "I think you are causing me to cough." How she knew this, we don't know; but she did. I opened my eyes, and Joan's hands were right in front of my nose and mouth. With amazement, I also knew this could be a possibility. I wondered how could I, a totally different person, be affecting Carolyn's physical body?

Joan then decided to set up her massage table, and asked Carolyn to lie down. I had the idea to pull up a chair and sit down beside Carolyn. As Joan hovered her hands about twelve inches above Carolyn's body, Carolyn's cough intensified, almost as if there was a gag over her mouth. Joan removed her hands and Carolyn calmed down. Again, Joan put her hands in place, and again the choking cough began. Joan immediately pulled her hands away. The third time Joan put her hands in place, the thought came to me that Carolyn and I should touch but not just anywhere. Carolyn should touch my lower back where all my pain had accumulated. I should touch Carolyn's chest area. This interaction reminded me of two electrical wires completing a circuit.

All these messages came to me simultaneously. This twin occurrence had been our common language with unspoken words. (i.e., one would get the **thought** and the other one would **take** action.) As Joan placed her hands for the third time, Carolyn's guttural cough immediately surfaced, full-fledged and very strong. I placed Carolyn's hand on my lower back, then placed my hand on Carolyn's chest. Suddenly, and I mean suddenly, Carolyn's cough stopped. With all our mouths wide open, we looked at each other in amazement. That cough never just stopped; it had **always** taken its full course.

None of us knew what had happened. Our curiosity led us to continue our exploration. I don't remember the details, but what we got from this was an initial awareness of the subtle effect of all surrounding energies. We also realized for the first time that Carolyn and I were more connected than we had ever thought possible. Our twinship was teaching us something about which we had no knowledge. We pondered our next step. The most significant clue we had was that Carolyn's energy was affected by a force just outside her physical body. I was affected by a force that entered or hit my physical body. What was this force, was it the same force, and what could we learn from it?

Joan explained the concept of "subtle bodies," wherein each one of us has not only a physical body, but emotional, mental and spiritual bodies as well. We had some prior knowledge about this, but there remained some yet unanswered questions. We perceived that some mysterious outside "force" was trying to bombard us. At that time, all we could understand was that Carolyn and I had a deeper metaphysical connection… and we didn't even know what that meant.

That night while sleeping, Carolyn awakened with a coughing attack, which was not unusual. She frequently had them at night. I went to see if I could assist her in any way. After about forty-five minutes, she appeared calm enough for me to ask if I could return to bed. She nodded yes. For some reason, the idea never occurred to me to apply what we learned earlier in the day with Joan.

Just as I was about to lay my head on the pillow, I had an eerie feeling that my life was going to change—I mean, really change!!! I heard Carolyn in the other room. She was in a full-blown attack, gasping for air. Immediately and simultaneously, we went to the kitchen to heat up some water. Hot water seemed to calm her aggravated airways.

I don't know why but, I began yelling. I wasn't yelling at Carolyn, but out of frustration I yelled to God, in a very loud and angry voice, "What the hell's going on here?"

No sooner did the words leave my mouth when an image of my mother appeared. Needless to say, I was in awe; but more importantly, I felt an enormous amount of peace surround my body. Her image was bigger than life itself. I felt my heart expand as love poured into it. The presence that she radiated could have knocked Carolyn and me down. Equally as important, I visually needed to **see** that my mother was no longer sick.

I looked at Carolyn with bewilderment and exclaimed, "Did you see her Carolyn? It was Mother. She was here!!!"

With a weakened and raspy voice, Carolyn said, "No, but that's Mom's presence. That's how she has come to me on so many different occasions."

I wondered if I was dreaming?

For the first time, I knew that there was something more to life than I had experienced. Mother's sudden presence (or was it an image of God using my mother's form?) was my first conscious wake-up call. Besides being awed by the experience, I felt an awakening deep in the core essence of myself. For the first time in my life, I felt aware and **present** in the experience of life.

Carolyn and I stayed up almost the rest of the night, talking about Mother's death and the night she died. This conversation led us to a depth of understanding that we had never shared before. As we talked, we realized no one had ever talked about Mother since she died. We each discussed how we thought Mother's death had affected us.

Carolyn didn't know why she had gone through so much grieving when I didn't feel that Mother's death had scarred me in any way. I felt as if my life had moved on.

We talked about the presence of Mother in the room.

We both knew our mother's presence--which was NOT foreign to us. We wondered if she wanted something from us, and if so, what? Her presence had scared us, but only because we did not know how to communicate with her. Carolyn told me that for years, when she would get really depressed, she often felt Mother around her. I told Carolyn that sometimes when I had my childhood accidents, I knew Mother was with me, too.

Were we crazy? If we had shared this with anyone else in our family, they would have thought that we were losing it. So, we not only kept it from others, we also denied Mother's existence from ourselves. Painfully we had kept our mother's visitations a secret. Now, we found comfort in each other's arms talking about our mother.

We went back to bed for a couple of hours before our late morning acupuncturist appointment. On the way there, I had the idea that Carolyn and I needed to be treated in the same room. The needles should be placed in her front and my back, almost as if we were one person. We asked the doctor if he would be willing to give it a try. How could we have explained it to him; we didn't even understand ourselves. He placed the needles in me first and then into Carolyn. Just as he left the room, I had another vivid image of Mother, seated right next to me. I saw the concerned look on her face, with the wrinkles in her forehead, and the color of her sweater. A cardigan with brown *and beige checks. It was all so real!*

I yelled to Carolyn and asked if she could see Mother. She said that she couldn't. I wondered why not??? Carolyn's the sick one. With that thought, I went into excruciating pain. I yelled to Carolyn for help. I thought I was going to pass out from all the pain.

"Feel the pain," Carolyn said, "and go into it."

"I wonder what the hell that means," I thought. Simultaneously, Mother got up and started walking out into the distance. With each of her steps, the pain subsided a bit more in my body. This went on, as if in slow motion, for the entire treatment. Then, suddenly, my mother looked at me and vanished. In that same instant, my pain of twenty-seven years (or a force of energy, as I call it now) had been lifted from me and vanished with her. I was stunned and elated all in the same second. (Hmm? I thought Mother's death had no visible impact on me. Guess I was wrong!)

The doctor removed our needles. I had no idea that my back pain and the death of my mother were connected. And now, I discovered that the pain in my back was the way I carried my grief over Mother's death. What did it all mean and why hadn't Mother freed Carolyn as well? My focus went from elation to concern. What about Carolyn?

We returned for one more acupuncture treatment the following day. I wanted to make sure that all my pain was gone.

I felt that I was truly given a gift from God, and a profound new life with a new body. From the time my mother first appeared, I kept my husband Terry informed about my transformation. He thought it incredible and didn't even question my sanity. He could tell by the tone in my voice that I was not the same Marilyn.

Carolyn and I had no one to guide us to our next step.

As we drove back to Atlanta, I joked to Carolyn, "I hope Mother doesn't show up in the car or on the windshield. I don't know if I could handle that one." We both laughed, but we knew we still needed answers for Carolyn.

We drove for about six hours. Marilyn was tired. It was getting dark and she didn't like to drive in the dark. We stopped to get her something to eat. I had just eaten the meal I brought along with me, and it was my turn to drive. Wrong! I began one of my coughing attacks, so I couldn't drive. I had to remain on the passenger's side with a paper bag because I often vomited during these attacks. Marilyn continued to drive. After two hours, she yelled, "What is all this about?"

I knew she wasn't yelling at me, and after she asked that question, the thought came to her that I should put my left hand on the part of her back that had given her a lot of trouble over the years. No sooner did we get our hands in position, my cough stopped. As we have stated before, my cough never just stopped, yet it had been doing just that a lot over the last couple of days. We were again amazed and full of questions. What were we being shown that we had no capacity to understand?

We had another piece to our puzzle; my previous back pain, Carolyn's cough and Mother's death were all related. We had been experiencing a triangular dysfunction with subtle bodies. But what did this mean, and what were we suppose to be learning? We continued with our drive, filled with questions about the future. Carolyn drove the rest of the way into Atlanta.

When we returned to Atlanta, we sought answers to all of our questions with the assistance of a hypnotherapist who understood metaphysics. We started to unravel what we discovered during the Florida trip, and received confirmation that Marilyn's back problems and my respiratory distress were indeed related and connected to the death of our mother.

Now, with the completion of our awesome six months, we can move forward in our dance to wellness. Needless to say, our lives were never going to be the same. We are sure there are other people who have had similar experiences to ours. What is unique about our wake-up calls is that we were gifted to stay awake so that we could assist in awakening the spiritual consciousness that is being stirred up on this physical plane.

What was amazing about that trip was that we drove straight through the whole eleven hours, and my back didn't even bother me. That was a major accomplishment for me because before my instantaneous healing, I couldn't sit for more than an hour at a time. When Carolyn dropped me off at my home, it was early morning. I tried to be quiet, but when I went into the bedroom, I woke Terry up. He couldn't believe his eyes. He wanted to touch my lower back immediately. He said there was a presence about me that he had never seen before and the lower part of my back, where it was always cold, was now warm. I got into bed and fell fast asleep.

The next morning I was still elated and high from our adventure. Unfortunately, Carolyn could not share in my elation. She was still at square one. We only had puzzle pieces. Carolyn was still physically slipping away.

Luckily, through my chiropractor, I knew two people who dealt with the paranormal. They offered their support, but said that the journey was only for Carolyn and me to experience and decipher. I needed help. Carolyn was still too sick to actually participate in these interpretations. At that time, I wondered why Carolyn and I weren't freed from our pains together since we were identical twins.

The next week passed quickly, full of new information. I felt bombarded and overwhelmed with thoughts that I felt were coming from my deceased mother. Had I really opened my communication with her, or had I imagined the whole thing? It really didn't matter. The one constant was that I felt alive and full of an energy that I had never before experienced.

I spoke with my dad several times about what had happened, including Carolyn's and my contact with Mother. I sensed from my father's reaction that he thought I might be losing my grip on reality. He even phoned Terry to ask how I was. My older sister also called Terry. He reassured them both that I was absolutely as sane as he had ever seen. (Terry was like E.F. Hutton…when he spoke, people listened.)

The conversations that opened up with my family were because of the actions I had taken under my mother's orchestration. I felt her presence and guidance so strongly it was even comical. I laughed as I found myself doing unusual things.

For instance, Carolyn called me early one morning. Mike was out of town, and I was on call. She was gasping for air and needed assistance. I ran right over, telling Terry I would return as soon as possible. Carolyn was only five minutes away, and as I drove to her, I got the thought, "You have to call your father." It was the middle of the night and I knew he was asleep, but the message was strong. I convinced myself to at least wait until 4:00 a.m. to call. My call awakened him, and I could tell he was not pleased. I spoke with him for a few minutes until he said, "Can I call you in the morning?"

"Yes," I said, and apologized for the time of day I had called.

I decided to stay with Carolyn, and thirty minutes later the phone rang. It was my father and this time he wanted to talk.

That was the start of us talking about our mother to our father. It was the beginning of opening up closed emotions we all had locked away deep inside of us.

My instantaneous healing and Carolyn's near-death experience allowed me to visually separate us and see us as two individuals; a separation I so desperately needed. I no longer needed to pull Carolyn around like "dead weight". We were freed and separated, and had experienced a new level of healing.

Carolyn's near-death encounter had a profound effect on me. Not only did I see a spirit come over her body and the force from her cough leave, but an insurmountable peace had entered my body. I also simultaneously felt my consciousness rise to a higher level.

On the physical level, my artistic talents exploded. The release from all my blocked emotions had taken a new form. I had toyed with some creative art endeavors while I practiced dental hygiene. I loved working with my hands. Cleaning teeth had been my creative outlet, but since I was no longer practicing dental hygiene, that energy needed another outlet. I never dreamed I was an artist.

We finally moved into a big house. We had lots of room and empty wall space. The first of my creative endeavors now appeared on canvas (instead of staying blocked within my body). I was pleased at how I was able to express myself with colors. It gave me such joy. I found old pieces of furniture that needed a new glow and gave them color. I used floor coverings on tabletops. I was like a puppy exploring the great outdoors for the first time.

You might wonder sometimes how to discover your own hidden talents. We all have them. It is our natural birthright to be joyful. It is natural to want to discover it. Unfortunately, my true self-expression had been stuffed into dormancy. I highly recommend to anyone who is stuck, just start painting. It's a lot of fun, and who knows what you might discover about yourself.

I always felt it was a mother's role to guide her children to creatively express themselves. In my case, I felt cheated. I didn't get that from my mother. I was angry and I stuffed that anger deep inside, which had prevented my creativity and joyful self-expression. There was no blame here, only me discovering myself.

For many years, Carolyn and I had our personal physical dramas and traumas. The reason that doctors could not totally help us was because they weren't looking at the whole picture. Of course, neither were we. The whole picture for Carolyn and me was that we needed to come together and heal as one. That may sound strange, but for thirty plus years we hadn't gotten to the bottom of our so-called problems. We had not been addressing them in the right manner.

As we continued researching and seeking out others to assist us in our quest for wellness, we gathered clues that were not the "norm". We had to make several shifts in our own beliefs and perceptions. With the appearance from my mother (actually five visitations in all) and Carolyn's near-death experience, God finally had our attention.

We were awake!

For many years I had been writing these memoirs about Carolyn's and my journey, thinking it was just for us and not for publication. Many times, after I felt that they were completed, these memoirs went back on my bookshelf. Each time I placed them there, I heard a small but very distinct inner voice say, "You have a message to share with others."

*It turns out that the night my mother died, my grief took the form of physical pain. Carolyn's grief manifested itself in depression, and later in respiratory illness. We all know when we are physically incapacitated, but Carolyn's respiratory affliction was her emotional self, crying out for attention. Through our journey, we have found that any illness stemming from the respiratory system, on a deeper level, is a manifestation of emotional needs not met. We have asked ourselves this question on many occasions, "Was Carolyn's cough only **her** cry for attention? Or, was she mirroring into me that I, too, had deep, uncried tears?*

Hindsight provides us with clues, and ours was no exception. We just needed to learn the language and interpretation. When I hit an all-time-low with my back pain, Carolyn began praying that she could help me in some way. Shortly thereafter, she got sick. It was as if her immune system broke down overnight.

The immune system talks to us in regard to "ourSelf". This is not simply about what's going on in our physical body, but how we feel about our physical body, our emotional body, our mental body, and even our spiritual body. It is all one and not separate. All our "selves" have to be in sync, or in harmony, with one another. If not, disharmony manifests, causing illness. Dis-ease. With Carolyn's and my situation, it was a little harder to identify. The bottom line was, we still needed to give "ourSelves" separate attention and distance, but that attention had to be in sync with the other one.

What Carolyn and I had to find out was, how did we both get so out of control with our pains? That answer would lead us to the why. Carolyn apparently took all the emotional pain over mother's death not only for herself, but for me as well (and maybe the rest of the family). And I had taken on that same grieving pain for both of us in the physical form (and maybe for the entire family). I say the rest of the family with question because we didn't really focus in on them. But what we also learned about the reason for this sharing of "stuff" was familiar. It was our way of being in the womb together. It was all we knew how to do. This sharing went as deep as cellular sharing, and we didn't have anyone to help us explore this connection.

One thing was for certain--Carolyn and I had been dancing this vicious cycle of sharing all our lives. And we were stuck. Once we recognized what we had been doing, one of us needed to lead us out of this pattern. I feel that's the role my husband Terry played when we got married. It was my first time of being around someone who was so healthy.

During this time, we often asked ourselves the question, "Did Carolyn get sick to help free me up from my physical pain?" We still don't know for sure, but one thing we found out--when it is time to wake up, it is on God's time, and not one moment before.

Carolyn and I discovered what that mystical bond between twins is. Simply put, it is shared energy. Some twins are more intertwined than others. We found that it doesn't just happen with twins, either. It can be between mothers and daughters, fathers and sons, husbands and wives, best friends, or even with someone deceased. When stuck, it is important to do your own detective work and find the missing "subtle energy" that will help free you up.

When someone is sick in a family unit, it is not just the sick person who needs attention. The whole family needs to work on freeing themselves in order to become the persons they were "meant" to be. This can be tricky. You can't "make" someone work on him or herself. What you can do is work on yourself, and pray that the other person receives the help they need. Carolyn and I found that as one of us healed at one level, the other automatically healed too. As we continued healing, we watched our family dynamics shift as well.

It was 1990 when I died and came back. Each day I get stronger. Each day I take time before getting out of bed to make sure I am connected with God in my thoughts. I have realized that I am a conduit of God's love. One of my purposes here on earth is to bring this awareness to others. I am no different than anyone else. I am but a conduit. I tell my clients you can be a con-do-it too. As we continue to connect to our Higher Power, and to discard the "baggage" of negativity from our minds, bodies, and souls, we are able to hold on to more of God's love.

However, this is not enough. We must learn how to both give and receive love. With me, this is a never-ending process.

I feel very blessed for going through my experiences. It was difficult at the time, but my illness led me to three major discoveries:

1)   How to get well and stay well.

2)   How to learn to let go of the negatives in my life...people, jobs, thoughts, and emotions.

3)   How to begin to live again...the desire to be well instead of sick.

As I said many times before, I grew up in illness and carried that dynamic forward in my life. I knew only how to be around sick people, or people looking outward to doctors for a cure. As I began to unravel my illness, I found fear behind it; fear of living, fear of being with other people, fear of others hurting me, fear of people leaving me, and fear of knowing myself. It is so easy to blame others. It is so easy not to take responsibility for oneself and I was an all-time master.

Many of us always put the needs of others before our own; everyone is so much more important. I did this very thing. Over the years I learned that if I continued to give to others and did not take time to replenish myself--to get quiet, to be in silence--then my body would again begin to cry out with the cough. I have learned that I am just like a baby--very delicate, but not fragile. If I forget to first take care of myself, I immediately stop, tell myself I am sorry, and go into silence to re-balance myself.

Through my illness, I learned that I had surrounded myself with other people who were ill. People who had also stopped their flow from life and having fun. I came to realize that I no longer wanted negativity in my life. I wanted people who were positive. I acknowledged that I could no longer be around certain family members. I realized I had to change the thoughts I had about others and myself.

Looking back, I can see that I brought myself to a point where I could no longer laugh or cry. Either release would set off a coughing attack. I learned to shut off these emotions, or so I thought. As I look back, I see that the coughs were my cries. I was purging my negativity, my pains, my sorrow, my grief that I had stored so deep inside.

I see that my house was a blessing. It was my school. Through my search I learned about subtle energy. This type of energy is not taught in standard textbooks.

I remember visiting a psychic, Barbie, in 1983, four years before my immune system broke down. She told me that I needed to get in touch with my metaphysical side.

I retorted, "What for? I'm having enough trouble with my physical side."

She was only a messenger. I had no idea what she was talking about. Neither did I have the curiosity to embark on a quest for more information. God gives us choices through different opportunities that have doors or windows we can use. I had an opportunity to open up, but at that time, I chose to keep that door closed. My metaphysical side had to wait.

By learning about subtle energies through my house, I transferred this knowledge over to my everyday life. As an identical twin, I saw how Marilyn's and my subtle energies affected one another.

We extended this awareness to include our spouses, and then our environments, and eventually our interactions within our environments. As I learned more about the Divine Plan, I realized how all of this affects our lives. At first I thought this line of thinking was somewhat "crazy"; but I learned to keep my mind open and continue expanding my awareness. I learned how the universal law of cause and effect plays out in our lives. What we think, we become. If we think in a negative manner (the cause) we may become ill (the effect of our thoughts).

Lots of people—doctors, psychologists and metaphysicians—are talking and writing about the power of our thoughts, along with our mind's ability to heal ourselves. One of my purposes is to bring to the foreground how these thoughts not only create our own realities, but also can affect the lives of our spouses, children, families, and friends. **Every** thought is heard, it has a domino affect.

What Marilyn and I learned on our journey, our journey of intertwinedness, is that people are connected. The unconscious thought of one person can create interference in the reality of another person. We also learned, with the assistance of our deceased mother, that people can still be connected, even though they are no longer on this physical plane.

Due to the interconnection with our mother when she passed over, our psyches did not want to let her go. I think that's why we created our bodily discomforts and illnesses. Unconsciously, it was our way of holding on. Neither one of us felt the closure we needed. We did not consciously do this, but we were not allowed to see her after she died, nor did we get to go to her funeral. These were circumstances we had unconsciously set up for ourselves to nudge us into "soul growth." We also learned that we were "open vessels," and because Mother had difficulty leaving this plane, she stayed connected with us through illness. Marilyn and I learned through our expanded awareness that the earth plane is where we come to learn lessons, feel emotions, learn to love and be loved, re-connect with God, and grow as souls. We heal from the inside out.

Another awesome result from Carolyn's and my experiences was our psychic abilities. We had always had a different form of communication as twins; our "sixth senses" were well developed. Our journey was about becoming aware of this sixth sense.

We as a people, the human race, have been healing our wounds from ancestor to ancestor. This is called "mass consciousness." As one person heals, it helps heal our families, our friends, our co-workers. Piece by piece, we gather the information needed to heal as a people. It's hard to see, and most of the time goes unnoticed, but this is what each one of us has chosen to come here to do.

The greatest time of mankind's evolution on this planet is now; consciousness is being expanded. More people than ever are searching for their own inner truths by seeking guidance from a power greater than themselves. More people than ever are connecting to their own "God within". This is neither a cult nor an epidemic. We are interdependent, and each one of us is finely tuned to the synchronicity of the Divine Plan. We just have to open up to the music. We are God's symphony!

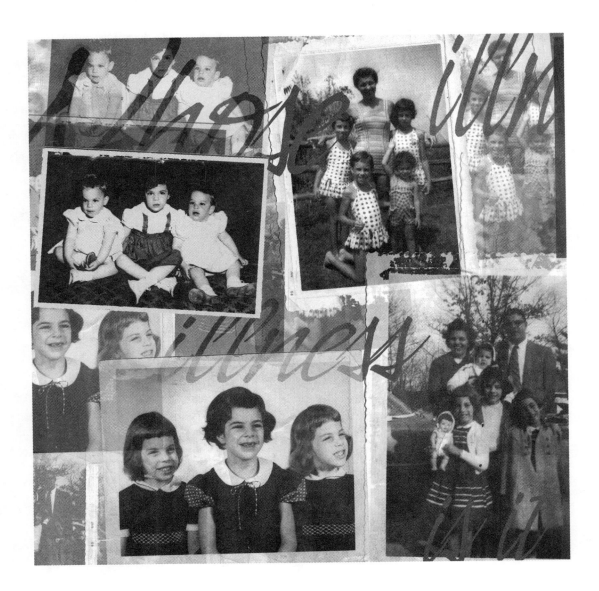

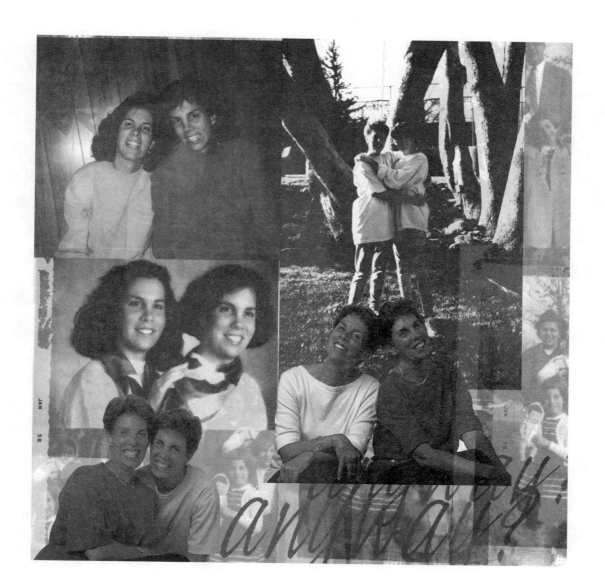

Part II

Untying the Knots

•**A reader's Note:** This section is written in Marilyn's voice. The typeface is not meant to distinguish between Marilyn and Carolyn as it did in the previous sections.

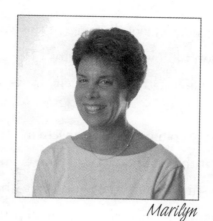
Marilyn

From Worrier To Warrior

*I*n my journey, I discovered that God had been working with me for years. There were many signs, but I was not open enough to read them. God was working through my mind, body and soul; however, my mind and body were disconnected. After my instantaneous healing, it was as if a light turned on and suddenly my SOUL was ready for growth. I could almost hear my soul scream with joy. I was hungry (no, starved) for knowledge. The issues that I had created were pretty painful. It was my way of shutting off the world while I grieved. The only problem was—I didn't know I was grieving. The emotional pain over my mother's death was so traumatic that I physically froze. That's why I was in pain for so long.

The issues that kept coming up for me were mostly physical. It never once occurred to me to look at the emotional or mental counterparts of my problem. Life has so many interesting dimensions, and what I had to learn was how to balance the physical, emotional, mental and spiritual parts of myself. In a nutshell, I had to find my own illuminated path and work in harmony with my mind, body and soul. I discovered that each and every moment, I had a choice as to how I could handle and/or react to my problems. My soul had been crying out for me to listen to it. My only hope was to work with my spirit. I wasn't aware of this side of true healing until it happened to me. I have called this the shadow side to my soul.

When I had my instantaneous healing, I KNEW immediately that there was a powerful force outside of me, and a love so huge that words cannot describe. It was the true beginning of allowing my desperate soul to work in unison with God in my physical form. Needless to say, my life was never the same. As I continued with a deeper search for myself, I was led into my "shadow self." I kept praying for more; and for a physical separation from Carolyn. I needed to put some distance between us. I knew that at some level, life could be lived even fuller than I had experienced. Carolyn was a large part of my life, and I was more than ready to explore my life separate from her. However, I didn't know that what I was praying for had so much fear attached to it. Shortly after I began praying for this separation, Terry got a job in North Carolina. Spirit had heard my pleas for help, and within a few short weeks I began the climb deep down into the wounds from my past.

As I surrendered to that shadow side of myself, I realized that this was a part of me that needed a voice. I knew I had been living a duality with Carolyn. What I had not grasped was the concept that I was whole all by myself. This may sound unusual to hear, but my fear kept me from knowing me. I knew Carolyn as somewhat the sadder twin and myself as more of the joyful twin. What I didn't realize was that in my "shadow side" were the emotions that I was afraid to explore. Does this make any sense? I was afraid to let down my guard, to feel grief or even sadness, because if I did, what would happen to my joy? Would my grief take me over? Would I begin to feel the sadness I always saw in Carolyn? I couldn't let that happen.

My prayers were already in action and I was moving forward just with the thought of wanting separation from Carolyn. Terry's and my move to North Carolina let me begin to remember what grief felt like.

In short, I got a "crash course" in grief. Leaving Carolyn was hard enough; but leaving Atlanta and my home and friends and all the things that were familiar to me was excruciating. I felt despair. I felt lost. All the emotions I had never wanted to feel were right there on the surface. I was definitely uncomfortable. I realized that this was not a great place to be, but was a much-needed place for me to explore.

At an even deeper level, I feared that if Carolyn expressed more joy in her life that would automatically push me to express my unhappiness. (I know this sounds silly, but our "twin-duality" often reflected the opposite. It's very interesting to experience this dynamic consciously.) I cannot express how fearful I was about the possibility that there might be a darker side to myself. What if I didn't like myself? As I moved through these fears, I realized I was okay. Emotions are just what they are, and like clouds, emotions, too, shall pass. Luckily I had good tools with which to work and had surrounded myself with highly skilled people who helped me embody and embrace my spiritual self.

This other side of me was foreign. The miracle that evolved from all this was that I learned that I am whole and separate from Carolyn. This may sound strange, but the shared energy between us was all I had ever known. It was time for both of us to be set free. If any of you have ever experienced a dependent relationship with another, it will be easier for you to identify with this concept. The miracle was that I was ready, willing and able to set myself free. The "shadow side" of self is the part of one that has no voice. It is the part of you that you keep hidden from yourself. It's the part of you that keeps resurfacing time and time again to be looked at and be healed. It's the part of you that screams to you mentally (with the negative mind chatter), emotionally (through depression, over-eating, drugs, alcohol, turmoil/unsettledness), and physically (through aches and pains in our bodies, or cancer, or other dis-ease). It is the part of you that is so frightened you start to question everything that you already have knowledge of, and become fearful to explore something new. The bottom line is downright fear. Fear is our "shadow side."

All my worries have unfolded to challenge me to become a warrior for myself. I have found that I am brave. Pain has been my teacher. As Carolyn's and my dance of personal pains continued to be our focal points (many times intertwined), something had to change. Neither Carolyn nor I ever dreamed that our missing link to wellness was the absence of our spiritual sides. I am not referring to my religious upbringing; that is a separate entity. Each of us had to discover our own relationship with ourselves and with Spirit.

As we look back on our mother's death, that pain kept us both locked in our past. Our bodies were the only thing that were in the present. It appeared as if Carolyn had been experiencing all the grieving over Mother through her depression. The flip side of that same coin was: What was I doing? Had I carried that same burden through my back problems? Carolyn and I were so used to sharing (all the way down to our sentences), that it never dawned on us to come together and heal as one person. When we finally did, we enabled each other to get to the root of our pains.

I cannot say that living without a mother has not been painful. It has been terribly painful. In my opinion, the mother is the most influential person on this planet. Her essence alone stands as the nurturer; a powerful role to undertake without full awareness of what that job entails. I think I will always have a lonely spot in my heart from the loss of my mother and the implications it has had on my life. I don't know what it would feel like to have a real mother; no different than not knowing what it would feel like not to be a twin. One thing is for sure, I am ever so grateful for all my learning experiences and the challenges I have had to overcome.

I was fortunate to have had three "mother" role models in my life. Unfortunately, though, I was unable to hold onto any of them and call them "mine." This is where part of the twist in Carolyn's and my relationship was overidentified.

We complicated our dynamics by reaching out to each other to replace our lost mother. We were afraid to move forward and petrified to let each other go. Will those dynamics ever change? They are still going on.

So, like any dance, our pains resurfaced time and time again. It wasn't until Carolyn was stricken with a life-threatening illness that we were able, with the help of Spirit/God, to move out of these roles and begin our new dance.

The best part about writing this story for me has been, with each re-read, getting more insights to propel me to another level. I get fresh new eyes with which to see myself from a different perspective. I get a clearer understanding of where I have come from, what emotions still have fuel behind them and need attention, and where I still need redirection in my life.

A new level of healing has been placed in front of me with our move to North Carolina. For the first time in many, many years, I have the chance to explore all of me. My shadow self, my big Self and my little self; I get to explore the whole me. I am coming into knowing myself, and that is a constant. I realize I am not just a person in human form, but a part of a more incredible whole picture. I am part of the universe, and that makes me a universal being. With the acceptance of self comes a huge amount of responsibility. With this responsibility comes sharing. The information I have received in my own learning needs to be shared. We all are gifted and have unique purposes in the Divine plan. **If we don't share with others what we learn, that new energy and information will be given to someone else to bring forward.** Information and knowledge guides each one of us into a higher level of consciousness. That's how we evolve as people and as a planet.

As I have continued to learn about myself, I have taught myself how to create my passions and desires with universal energy and bring it down into physical form. This has been a gift that I received from God through my healing experience. I am constantly learning HOW to use this energy, WHAT to do and what needs to change. It's important for me to continue fueling my passions with this "fire energy" I access and utilize from the universe. This fire energy has always been inside me, but through misuse and lack of guidance, I used this energy to create my pains. I do take full responsibility for this misuse, I do not blame it on stupidity, rather on the lack of my conscious exposure.

The question I have to ask myself is: What was I worried about and what was I fighting? Within my own family dynamics, I was fighting with my sister, Natalie, who I felt bullied me. In the same breath, and at a very deep level, I hear a small, faint voice inside my head say, "I was worried that people wouldn't like me because I didn't have a mother." That was from my inner child's perspective. I didn't want people to see me as different. I wanted to be a warrior and feel strength.

In reality, my foundation was broken. I felt that my support had been robbed. I encourage myself to probe even deeper and look at what is underneath all this.

Again, another faint voice inside my head says, "There's no one leading the family. There's no one here to protect me or guide me. I feel lost. I feel scared."

I was in the duality of not wanting anyone to see my pain; yet, I desperately wanted someone, anyone, to reach out and lift my heart to safety.

From a very early age I learned how to protect myself. I began withdrawing from family members who I thought were harming me, either with unkind actions or with harsh ugly words. I appeared cold and non-participatory to others. But what I was really doing was dimming my light so no one would notice my intense pain.

The Beat Goes On

I felt very fortunate and blessed to have had my wake-up calls, but I was confused as to how to proceed with the writing of this book. I knew I was finished writing about my past. As far as the present, everytime I tried to expand on who I was, I only found an empty feeling with a huge void. I think it is very important to heal from the past, and at times it is necessary to keep going over it. But when does one shut the door on it and move on? I decided that the time was NOW, and for the first time in years, I became ready to bring this project to completion.

What I now want to offer to you, the reader, is who I am today; and how healing, at all levels, is so very important. As I heal, my awareness is expanded and my connection to the Divine is strengthened. My part in God's scheme is to raise consciousness. By sharing myself and setting an example, I hope I have done just that. Life is a journey presented in lessons, and a serious lesson is about "lightening up." As Richard Carlson says in his book, **Don't Sweat The Small Stuff...**"It's *all* small stuff."

I wanted to get to the "meat" of who I was becoming, and everyday I looked forward to the process of watching myself unfold. Before I explain the process of my own unfolding, it is important to point out that when you are ready to do **your** work, be prepared. I was absolutely not prepared to fall as low as I needed to go in order to get back up.

I had been praying for a new direction in my life. I wanted a better relationship with Carolyn, my other sisters and my father. I was tired of conducting these relationships in the same way...from a distance (except with Carolyn). Our relationship, on the other hand, was the opposite--too close and intertwined. All I knew was I wanted things to be different, and I had an intuitive feeling that they could.

My prayers were answered when Terry was offered a job in Charlotte, North Carolina. That was doable. Charlotte was only a few short hours away from Atlanta and had a very similar climate. Terry and I visited Charlotte for the weekend to check the city out before he accepted the job.

That night, I learned in my dreams that this pending adventure was going to be emotionally and mentally challenging for me. I had never experienced such an explicit dream. On a conscious level, I was experiencing terrifying fright. I had the feeling these emotions were coming from somewhere in the distant past, yet

I could not relate them to my life. It felt strangely like fear from my life in another time—the 17th Century! I knew about past lives, but I was certainly not consciously prepared to go into one. I even told Terry the next morning that if he took the job, it was going to be a rough journey for me.

Every emotion raced through my mind. I was excited! Scared. Exhilarated. Confused. Not wanting to leave Carolyn behind. Angry—yet I felt gutsy and very eager to take this plunge.

Within two months, I was living in Charlotte. Within a month after that, my positive attitude took a rapid dive. I had prayed to God before leaving Atlanta that I wouldn't lose the good things I had developed, such as my evolution in consciousness. I was scared that I might go back to "sleep." That's what I was afraid was happening to me. I felt as if a veil was covering the new me that I had worked so hard to get to know. I got angry. I was angry with God. I was angry with Terry, and I was angry with myself. I was angry with my realtors for selling me my house. I was angry in the house. I felt as if we had bought the wrong house. I was prepared to move. I hit an emotional rock bottom.

This was in the fall of 1997. By Thanksgiving, I politely (that's how I am—never wanting to hurt anyone), honestly and bravely told Terry that I was afraid for our relationship. I felt I was being pulled by a very strong force that was spiraling me downward, and I had no one with whom to talk. I knew that all of Terry's energies were invested into his new job. I didn't want to seem selfish for his attention, but I was drowning. Interestingly, right after that realization, I felt that a huge secret burden had been lifted from me. I knew I needed to see a therapist. I also knew the therapist had to be an evolved, consciously aware individual who could understand and assist me on my journey. I am always amazed at the rapidity with which the universe (spirit) responds to my needs. Very soon, I was given the name of a therapist from my veterinarian's sister. I placed a call, but it took me a couple of months to submit and allow myself to see her. I really thought I could do this alone. I was so used to doing things in this manner—on my own, independent, no mother, absentee father, no need for help from others —my old pattern. Little did I know that the old pattern was going to dissipate and I was on my way to a deeper level of healing and understanding myself.

My intention in seeking help was to learn to sort out my feelings. I was caught between the desire to return to Atlanta to be with Carolyn and a need to develop a separate, individual self. I was grieving deeply and very confused. I also felt other energies around me. I felt that the devastation from Hurricane Hugo (ten years earlier) was still present in Charlotte, and in my house. Maybe that was part of what I was feeling. (Have you ever had an eeire feeling that you were experiencing something that was out of your realm of comprehension? Well, this was one of those times.) It didn't matter; these emotions felt like mine, and it was I who had to deal with them.

One of my daily rituals has always been to write about what goes on and how I feel about it during each day. It's interesting because upon re-reading one's own writings, a lot of the "real you" appears.

It turned out that not only was I depressed; but also the house was pulling the depression out of me through its colors. I didn't resonate with the colors in the house. Not a problem, you might think; but I was battling two personalities and getting very confused. (This has been the story of my life!) The past owner's first name and mine were the same-Marilyn. The colors that were in my new home were really the colors Carolyn liked. The confusion left me paralyzed and unable to take the appropriate actions to move me to my next step. My whole life my father's friends called us Carolyn/Marilyn, Marilyn/Carolyn; and they still do. I was suddenly faced to deal with my confusion. How did my life get so confused? Did I bring this on myself? Where did I begin to lose myself? Was this confusion brought on by society (peers, family, teachers)? Carolyn and I were trapped in this confusion; that is why we stayed so caught up with each other's illnesses. Nevertheless, it was a behavior that had been imbedded into us. The healing would only take place if the behavior was identified and changed. I was now in the process of discovering my separation from Carolyn, and it was very scary. What if I had been depressed all my life and didn't know it because Carolyn had taken that "wrap" for me? I was spiraling downward and no one could help me, but me.

I knew colors healed. I had gotten in touch with that during my healing process in Atlanta. I was not aware of how colors can also pull out depression. Colors are a vibration, and so are we. There are so many hues and intensities to each color, all vibrating at different levels. The past owner, Marilyn, had decorated her house with colors that were more in harmony with Carolyn. I think I was angry because I felt that the house was really for Carolyn. I truly believed that God had gotten us mixed up. She was the one who had wanted to move. I loved Atlanta. I wanted to stay there, where I had already created a wonderful house. I knew how important a healing house was for my psyche. However, I had asked God to move me to my next level. I just didn't know the next level would be the healing of grief and depression; things I had never really felt before.

As my depression continued, I couldn't find enough energy to reinvent my new home. I was stuck in that energy. As hard as it was at first, through my past learning, I was able to recognize that this house was healing me. Recognition is the first step in healing; but how long would I stay down, and what was I supposed to be learning?

My challenges were in full play. Needless to say, that turned out to be an understatement. All of my buried anger needed to come up. It was if I had been placed in Charlotte to feel my anger. In an odd sort of way, I felt as if my life had been suspended in time and space, just so I could begin to heal my past emotional pains. I knew I was in a healing crisis. As hard as it was, I knew there would be light at the end of this dark tunnel. I often wondered how long this was going to take. On an even grander scale, I knew everything was in God's hands and I would move forward when He decided and not one second before.

Luckily, my prayers were answered and our time was cut short in Charlotte. We were only there for eighteen months. It was long enough to discover the real me and explore my emotional wounds consciously. I began to fit the pieces of my life back together. I had felt emotional disharmony in our family all my life, and had needed to sort my emotions out from everyone else's.

As I continued to play out my dynamics, by Thanksgiving 1998 we finally came together as a family to heal. I provided the space, and for the first time in over twenty-five years, my family got together and enjoyed each other's company. My stepfamily did not join us, and as hard as that was for my father, it was a much needed time for us to come together.

During those months in Charlotte, I came to understand myself, my past, and where I was going in my life from a much better perspective. I have more compassion for myself. I have learned to embrace all of me. I am all I've got. So I'd better like all of me.

I have always known about the disharmonies in my family, and I recognize that this disharmony started long before our stepfamily joined us. The bringing together of these two families just intensified what was already present. We reflected into each other what needed attention. The trouble was no one wanted to look at the dirty laundry. I don't think that we are the only dysfunctional family on the planet.

I believe that God is working with us from a higher place so we can go through these hardships in order to bring more peace and love into our hearts. All that is expected from us is that we do our own work. End of story. And when you look back over your years, you can "WOW!" yourself, because you took part in bringing more love to this earth.

We will discuss families and stepfamilies a little later, but before moving forward, I want to continue sharing my exploration as a "singleton." Remember, to me, becoming a singleton means finding healthy emotional boundaries, free and independent from Carolyn.

Going To My Next Level...
Exploring Life as a Singleton

*T*he most frequently asked question of Carolyn and me is, "What's it like being a twin?" (You can't imagine how many times we have been asked this question.)

My comment is always the same, "I don't know, I've never been a singleton."

I/we came into this life as a double. After high school, we split up to explore life as individuals, and not as a "we." Only, then, we weren't conscious that our separation was for any particular reason other than having different interests. In 1981, we came back together to unfold our mystical journeys to wellness. Our illnesses kept getting passed back and forth between each other. This was no different than a common cold being passed around in a family, workplace or school. Our journeys lead us down different roads, only to cross over and tie neatly into a knot, the mystical aspect of self, and lead us comfortably into the hands of

God. In a nutshell, our physical bodies were lacking the missing ingredient to become whole; that ingredient being God. A spiritual door had been opened and nothing in our lives was ever going to be the same. Funny, during my earlier years some of my friends became "born-again Christians," and I often wondered, "What's a nice Jewish girl like me have in store with God?" I never took those thoughts any further, and anyway, I already had my own life's dramas and traumas in play. I did have a few conversations with my dad, questioning religion in general. End of spiritual pursuit.

Well, God never gives up and is always reaching out to love you, even when you don't know it. That was one of my first lessons on God. After our "wake-up" calls came in, I was starved for more. I read anything and everything to help uncover myself to the deeper me. Years have gone by since the "calls" came in, and as I continued unraveling the real me, I always asked for my next lessons to be brought forward. As the old adage goes, "Be careful of what you ask for, you might get it!"

My next step in the healing of my mind, body and soul was to experience what it felt like to exist on a daily basis without Carolyn in view. I felt elated, yet very scared to take this step; but on a deeper level of consciousness, I knew it was a mandatory lesson.

Before Terry and I moved, I had a long talk with God and told Him that my biggest fear about moving was the fear of losing my connection to Him. I had grown so much in consciousness, and what I feared most of all was a veil of darkness engulfing me. That veil was fear. (How I was going to play it out was being unfolded for me.) I was afraid I would lose the new Marilyn I had uncovered; the one that felt safe and very loved.

The move was an easy one in regard to the movers packing us up and getting us to our destination. I visually couldn't see Carolyn every day, even though I knew we could talk on the phone. The distance to her house was in driving range if I really felt the urge to hop in the car and go "see" her. I said the move was easy; however, the transformation was not. My elation didn't last long, and that scared inner child soon surfaced. My "shadow side", the side I was always afraid to know, hit me head on. Within just one month, I hit the lowest point in my life; I hit depression.

Yes, this *was* getting repetitive. Read on.

What was this depression telling me? Did "it" have a language that I could understand? Reflecting back, now, I can see my fear was being masked by my depression. I also know that all the judgments I had placed upon myself, and probably Carolyn, were surfacing to be recognized so I could make the conscious decision to change some ugly behaviors. It never surprises me HOW the universe keeps putting the same lessons in front of us to get. In my terminology, judgment is the polarity we play out in our lives. Always trying to prove that we are right and that the other one is wrong. That force of push and pull sets into motion a negative reaction, and in my case with Carolyn, a very strong conflict. I was in search of making these necessary behavioral changes.

At first I assumed that the depression was from some of the work I had been doing with Carolyn. I had been so wrapped up in her problems that I thought they were just oozing from my pores. With time, I thought that it would pass. Days went by; some good, some not so good. I forced myself to get up and get going. I meditated. I took walks. I played ball a lot with my dog, Samantha. It was important for me to keep myself moving.

Terry was traveling more than we had anticipated, so I took the first opportunity to run back to what I thought would be the safety of Atlanta. My first visit there lasted only a day and a half. My old home, where I had once felt safe and happy, had been bought by Carolyn and Mike. That place I envisioned in my mind and heart no longer existed. That scared me, and I quickly ran back to my new home in Charlotte. I felt for the first time that I had no safe place to call my own. For the first time in my life, all my childhood fears were surfacing, begging for understanding and healing. It was time for me to really feel my buried emotions.

You might ask yourself at this time, "Why didn't I fix the house up and adjust it to suit my/our taste?" I'll answer that with this statement, "I was going to do so, but then I stopped." I wasn't sure if I liked the house enough to fix it up. I wasn't even sure if I wanted to stay in Charlotte at all. I wasn't sure of anything. The only thing I was sure of was that I was GRIEVING and scared, so I just froze. It was time to deal with my stuff.

Another thing I had learned shortly after moving was that I was going through menopause. This was not a fantastic time to move! I was dealing with the emotional side of myself, plus, I had no idea that these emotions were exacerbated by the hormonal mood swings that occur with "the change." I knew I had taken the plunge into the darkest side of myself, and I didn't know if I would come out smiling or not.

Before hitting this emotional island, I had mastered many spiritual tools. God talked to me daily, if not moment to moment. I really needed some tangible help on this earthly plane. I needed therapy; not just a good therapist, but one who could help me bridge my two worlds.

Luckily, no sooner had I asked for help when I was led to a woman who has since helped me work miracles in my life. **Again, the Universe supplied for my need.** Naturally, I was ready and eager to do any work she suggested. She said

I was very easy to work with because I was prepared for my sessions. She helped me learn to sort my feelings out about what I had been experiencing from only KNOWING and BEING a twin. She helped me begin to set healthy boundaries for myself with Carolyn. It was a natural response for me to consider another person's feelings before myself. I always thought that was being courteous. What I learned in therapy, though, was by putting others first, I put myself second, third, or even last. I had to recognize that I was still using behaviors from my childhood that no longer served me. I had outgrown them. A young woman raised by a father is at a disadvantage, in the sense that there is a special nurturing that only a mother can provide her children. My dad did his best, but NOW it was time to develop a little discernment for myself.

My "shadow side" of unfelt emotions still needed to be felt. Ouch! They stung. Consciously, I knew I was going through it; and luckily I knew what it was like to feel happy. When one has a foundation of happiness, it is easier to find your way back. It was just a matter of time.

I also needed a game plan. In my first book, THE HEART SPEAKS, I wrote about making a happy list. I meant it. We all make shopping lists, but how often do we even think about making a list of what will make us happy?

One of the reasons I started seeing a therapist was to help me figure out what I was going to do. Was I going to stay in Charlotte with Terry, or move back to Atlanta? I wanted a female therapist to help me learn to figure these and other things out, as I had never felt comfortable doing this. I was aware that either road I took would be a road to discovering "me" at a deeper level. All my life I had primarily gotten input from my father, and now I mainly consulted with my husband. I was searching for a good, old-fashioned "earthy" female to provide me with the female perspective that I had never learned. I intuitively knew that a female would encourage me to trust my intuition; my heart.

After only a few months of working with Kevin, my female therapist, the answer I had asked for evolved so naturally. I sat down and made up a game plan (with God, of course) and wrote this plan down. I shared it with Terry. It was doable. The plan was simple. I would "reinvent" only two of the rooms in our house: the kitchen and one of the bedrooms where color from the wallpaper greatly offended me.

Unfortunately, the house had a lot of wallpaper that had been playing havoc on my psyche. I knew that if I could just make these simple changes, I would be in a better frame of mind to plan out my next steps. I also knew that since I spent a lot of time in the kitchen, it made sense to give it the first make-over.

The rest of our game plan went like this: I would return to Atlanta while the room renovations were being made. Because I was still in the midst of my therapeutic "emotional sorting," I felt a deep need for my Atlanta refuge. Terry and I prepared ourselves for the possibility that if the renovations did not go well, he might have to make a commute back and forth. His job involved more travel than we had previously anticipated, so moving back to Atlanta was not a big issue. I had not planned to make any geographical changes until the year was up. All I was doing was trying to buy some time so I could emotionally raise my spirits enough to make an intelligent decision. Just in case, I had prepared myself for the worst case scenario. The most important thing at this point was to establish a continuation of Terry's and my game plan, and talk it over with him straight from my heart.

To my surprise, over the next few weeks, the house took on a beautiful transformation. I knew this was a symbolic sign from the universe that "IT" was working with me. (I just smile when I know I am connecting.)

About two weeks into the reinventing of my home, I was in a therapy session. I was telling Kevin about all the "stuff" that had been transformed, not only in my home, but in my family life, too.

She interrupted me and said, "It looks like you have made the decision to stay."

Without knowing it, I was preparing myself to remain in this house. Under all my erratic behavior was a deeper level of emotions that I kept buried deep inside. I had been aware of this all along, but I was not equipped to handle what was coming up for me. I was now in a new place with a lot of old feelings. I was definitely in a crucial pivoting point. Isn't this what transformation is all about? I had been afraid for my life because I knew my well-being was in jeopardy. My psyche was not strong enough to feed my emotional body with positive energy. I knew if this pattern of thinking continued for any length of time, my physical health would decline. I also questioned how my marriage would withstand this emotional roller coaster. (Isn't it funny, not only was I re-inventing my house, I was re-inventing me. Life has so many parallels.)

When I had first asked God to help me get to my next step with Carolyn, I had never dreamed that fear, pain and repressed emotions would be the next step. I was not prepared. However, in reality, we are always prepared. God doesn't give us anything that we cannot handle. My next step from Carolyn was to explore what it's like to be a singleton. Carolyn and I had been so very involved in each other's lives for so long, we didn't know where one boundary ended and the other began. That's what part of this transformation was all about.

The part of me that needed the most attention was determining how I should fill my days. I desperately needed to go through my depression and begin to heal the grief and loss issues for my mother. Loss had played a major role in my life. As strange as this might seem, "loss" was somewhat of a comfort zone. I knew it was time to move ahead and beyond these familiar feelings. In order to do so, I needed this valuable time to feel, heal, and fill. What I began noticing was that on some days I experienced this huge feeling of aloneness. No, it was not loneliness. I had to constantly check in with myself and ask HOW I was doing. I began to notice that this "aloneness" was just me finding myself without Carolyn. Being a twin is a unique experience. Energetically I can always feel Carolyn. That is an "is-ness" that will never change.

For the first time ever, I began exploring consciously what it was like to be me. Pretty exciting! Scary! You name it. It was definitely a brand new feeling; much like if you suddenly discovered you had an identical twin. I questioned many times if this aloneness had anything to do with God. From the heart level, I knew God was walking me through all this. I just had no clue as to what this "new me" was like, or what I was evolving into. I was shifting myself into a new way of being; one I had no reference point from which to gauge my transformation.

After my house was completed to a comfortable level, I knew it was time to get to the "real" reason as to why I was in Charlotte. For the first time in many years, I felt quiet enough to really sit down and write. I am supposed to be writing and sharing this journey with others. I asked God, and myself, "Why the wake-up calls?"

I heard a soft whisper in my head, "If I didn't knock you off your feet, you'd still be doing the same old thing." I like to interpret that to mean I would not have gone on searching and reaching for my higher truths. Physically, I was searching to get out of pain. But I was missing the main ingredient to getting well. I think we always have similar problems throughout our lives, but with each situation, each problem, it only takes us to a higher level of awareness and understanding. That, all by itself, takes our essence to a higher level of being.

As I move ahead, I must take the time to say that I am ever so thankful to be conscious enough to be thankful. I have come to recognize my gifts as a person on this planet. I am truly blessed with the abundance that each day brings. It's like a present waiting to be unwrapped. I never considered myself a great dental hygienist, but I was. In my past, I carried a lot of self-doubt. I learned I was good because I did the best I could. I taught each of my patients something new, and each one of my patients truly got a piece of my heart.

When I was searching for another career, I never dreamed that I would be doing what I am now. I always thought I would practice dental hygiene. But as life has it, there's always another opportunity looking straight into your face. I had already gained knowledge on how to work with the body, using my own body in the learning process. I loved working with people, and I had a lot of hands-on experience by being a twin and developing my extrasensory perceptions. By gathering this information and combining these gifts, I have opened up to what was already inside of me. That was just the beginning.

As I further allowed myself to open and blossom as a singleton, I discovered I had many talents that I was just beginning to tap into. The burst of colors came forward effortlessly. I started on canvas and moved myself onto furniture pieces. It was natural for me to want to transform everything that was in front of me. What I learned during this process was that colors heal. Colors, like the weather, affect our moods. I found it very necessary for me to stay in a certain color vibration in order to stay happy. That's why, when I moved my emotions took a dive. My intentions were to change the colors in my house immediately, but if I had, I wouldn't have had the experience of learning how to pull myself out of a downward spiral. Now I can pass this knowledge and wisdom onto others who experience depression, and teach them how to raise their vibrations and moods to another level. It's not just about shifting the vibration temporarily, it's about raising the vibration up to a level that is a happier one, and keeping it there. Colors not only affect how you feel, they also affect the way you eat and digest. Noise affects the way you eat and digest, too. I mention these tidbits because I thought it a good opportunity to pass it along. There's so much knowledge oozing out of my pores.

I began to develop my writing skills, (which I highly recommend), when I was in my healing process. I discovered the value of a daily ritual. Writing daily helps me tap into and solve problems that I do not easily understand. It helps me see me more clearly. I am just putting down what my skills are for now. I know that one of my precious gifts is that I am in tune with energy. Being a twin, I know nothing else. But I've taken this gift and developed it further. Using my intuitive abilities and my knowledge of the body, and combining it with feeling energy, I know I am developing these gifts for a reason. I say that loosely because this is developing into a spiritual movement for others. I love telling people about my wake-up calls. I don't know if I do it for shock, for some other type of reaction, or if I do it just to get other people to think about the "what-if's." What if there was more to life than what we are seeing? Could there be more? What would it be like if we all could tap into the "more"? I like to get others to begin to think differently and question their own lives. I'm not out to sell anything, just to bring awareness to others. Isn't that what life's about?

The more I began feeling a separation from Carolyn, the more I realized

I have had a lot of accomplishments. Funny, when you are a twin, you don't always see yourself clearly. Charlotte provided me the space to slow my life down, almost to a halt. I began to see myself more clearly; to really see HOW my life had been playing out. What aspects of my life needed attention. What needed to be set free. That included people, places and things that no longer served me for my highest good. Charlotte is a very family oriented community. Just by being in that environment, I was able to remember some deeply buried happy times. Until then, my heart had only remembered the painful ones. I joined the YMCA so I could exercise and swim. To get to the pool, I had to drive down a graveled road, go underneath big old trees, to where the pool was situated on top of a hill. Just with the drive to the pool, my senses were immediately transported to my childhood and happy times with my family, before my mother got sick. It was my most treasured hour of the day. I would sit and watch the mothers and their children play in the water. I was a part of that pleasure, and at the same time, I was able to get in touch with my sadness; my sadness of not having my mother. Feeling emotions and allowing them to be there is very healing. A part of me felt very empty. As I look back on it—empty is good, because it's a space you give yourself to fill with something positive. I not only felt empty without having Carolyn around, I felt empty for not having my mother too. It was my first time ever to feel this emotion. I needed to find this space so I could fill it with the people and things that brought me joy.

Charlotte became like a giant magnifying glass that I could look through to see how engulfed I had become in Carolyn's life. My world was too small!! I did not do this intentionally; our life's dramas and traumas caused us both to shut out life. It was now my time to start re-living. By being alone, I began refilling my days with people and things that mattered. I met new people. I began to allow people to love me. I re-opened my heart to my first stepmother, Roberta. It felt great! She had already come back into my life a couple of years before. I now lived a little closer to her, and she came to see me more frequently. She met my friends. She helped me with my house. Just by her reaching out to me when I needed it the most was enough. I know her presence made my separation from Carolyn more tolerable. I was reaching for more love, to be loved, to feel love, and God knew it and provided me with the people who were reaching back.

My world was being re-filled, and I was consciously participating. Charlotte had served its purpose. On the flip side of that same coin, I was still living in a place that did not resonate with me. I found out later, after we moved back to Atlanta, places and things are like people. There is a relationship going on, and if it doesn't feel right, no matter how hard you try, there are times when things just don't work out. I had to ask myself the question, "If my life were on hold, or if I were suspended in life for whatever reason—would I want to be spending it in Charlotte?" The answer was undoubtedly "NO!" It was time to move on. The end of my healing crisis was finally over. Thanksgiving was the event that needed to take place for me and my family, and it happened. It was time to go home.

Atlanta was my home, and just by me saying to Terry, "It's time to go home," was the healing my heart needed. I learned I did not want to move back too close to Carolyn. I needed a little space between us so I could remain independent from her and develop new friendships. I wanted my world to continue to grow. I found I needed to change old patterns of behavior. I wanted to send out good messages through my actions. That takes constant monitoring. God gives us each moment to act or react, and then gives us the next moment to correct it. Isn't that great? We are all creatures of habit, and I can honestly say I had some behaviors that were not pleasant. I am always going to be a work – no, I shall say, a masterpiece in progress.

For those who wonder HOW Terry went with this flow and the moving around, he was right there by my side. From the time we let Carolyn and Mike have our condo, Terry just allowed me to do whatever I needed to do. I know I am blessed because there are not many men who would put up with their wife's entanglement with her sister. I also know being married to a twin is an adventure all in itself.

Ways of Being

There are so many ways of being. You can be angry. Or you can be happy. You can't be both at the same time. Nor would you want to. To get full enjoyment from the emotions you are expressing, you must be present. A lot of times we live our lives by acting out past emotions and events. I know I have been guilty of that on numerous occasions. What was important for me to find out for myself was to know "me". That's what exploring life as a singleton let me examine. I wanted to get into my true essence. I had already been exploring "me" through my writings and artwork. But I still wanted to know what kind of vibration I was sending out. Do you ever wonder what vibration you are sending? I know certain people turn me off, and I know I turn some people off too. I was curious enough to learn more about what kind of vibration I was sending out, and how to work with it in a whole new light.

Everything has a vibration, and that vibration is in the form of energy.

You know how much better you feel emotionally when the sun is out. And how during the winter months, you feel blue when the sun doesn't shine for several days. When I started therapy, I was emotionally drained. I only had one way to go, and that was up. But I didn't know how to get up. After a few months of therapy, and with much praise from my therapist on how the work I had been doing was moving me forward by leaps and bounds, I asked my therapist what she really thought of me. A pretty loaded question. Was I prepared for her response? To my amazement, she told me as distraught as I was, underneath it all she felt my true essence of joy. I was so glad to hear that because that was who I thought I really was. I do express myself joyfully. Being joyful is my inner connection with the Divine energy. I also am aware that not everyone is comfortable being around someone who is happy. (Remember that being happy is a vibration.) I found that out when Carolyn was sick. Sometimes Carolyn would say to me that I was "too much" for her to be around. That was a very important lesson for me, because now I know to sort of bring my "wings" in when I am around someone who is sick. It's just learning to be considerate and courteous of another human being who's vibrations are struggling to come back into balance. I probably learned to withhold my joyful energy as a child by being around my mother. Children are prime examples of joy. They know no other way to be. It is our birthright to be happy. It's just that as we grow older, we get our hearts buried in all the "muck" from our life's dramas.

Through my separation from Carolyn, I have recognized we really do have different personalities. Our essences are different. I applaud myself for finally being able to see and feel that. It has freed us both up to fly. I am not afraid to be happy. I used to worry too much about others who were not happy. I felt it was my job to make them happy. Pretty exhausting work! I found out through my own healing that the other person who was consumed with worry, or fear, or depression was keeping present company with themselves. It was their way of being. Don't you feel that when someone is depressed or feeling down, they want to "unconsciously" pull you into their misery? Remember the old adage, "misery loves company."

As you begin opening your hearts up to more love and happiness, you'll start choosing who you want to spend time with. Listening to the news and reading about all the problems in the world, or your own city, leave you with negative thoughts and a negative vibration, let alone a negative feeling. And it leaves you to question who you really are. I know for myself, I always felt the world around me was a reflection, to some part, of my personality. (Must have been an inherited twin-concept or something.) Learning to become a "singleton" has allowed me the luxury of remembering that not everyone and everything is a reflection of me. Maybe I am supposed to be a thorn to someone else for his or her growth. But on/in the grander schemes of life, we all play a part of the whole. And yes, the action from another person does have a ripple effect on each and every one of us. I think that during Carolyn's and my healing process, we became living examples of this truth. So it's important to feed your psyche with positive information. Feed your bodies with nurturing foods. That's how one evolves into a higher state of being.

Learn to be responsible for your own self.

I have become very particular about how I want to spend my day. I have some rituals with which I begin each day. For instance, upon waking up each morning, I like to take time, just in case my dreams are trying to tell me something of importance, to quietly listen to my thoughts. Then my thoughts go to re-aligning myself with God. I like to bring all my energy fields back into alignment with me. I bless my day and ask God for a few favors, and tell Him what I want to accomplish for the day in order to walk my talk. I really try and pay attention to HOW I might appear to those that come in contact with me. I then meditate for about thirty minutes by listening to my breath. I stretch for awhile doing yoga and then I shower. I eat breakfast and go for my morning walk, getting in tune with nature.

And then the tone of my day is set. That's how I "be": I "be" by beginning. And everything else that happens for the rest of my day is a blessing. I am so fortunate to have the luxury of this lifestyle. I also know that this is my work. For a long time, I was consumed on what to do in my next career. I wanted to earn a good income. What I had to come to terms with was...I am doing my work. And the payoff is BIG.

Awakening the Body...

One needs to awaken the mind, body and soul. So get yourself moving!!!

How does one awaken their body? I wrote this section because this is where I was stuck. It is important for me to keep my body's energy flowing. I know mine was asleep for a very long time. But earth time is a lot different than spiritual time. Remember when you were a kid and the school year lasted for what seemed like forever? When I was stuck in my physical pain for twenty-seven years, that "stuckness" kept me caught between two focuses--the present with my physical complaints and the past with emotional pains. I was unconscious as to what I was thinking or with whom I surrounded myself. I was just plain "stuck." But in that brief moment of being set free, it was as if all those years vanished. It was like they never happened to me. It was as if freedom had been with me always. Does this make any sense? I write about this because no one ever told me that I didn't have to live like this. I want you to know that the mind is what holds you back. Delve into your pains. Ask what's underneath all of it. Go gently. Don't be afraid to go into your darkness. There is only light at the end of the tunnel. My light was God's light. Each of us has to explore that inner growth all by our "self." Where am I going with all this?

Start dancing. Get yourself moving. Blocked energy has to be moved out. What if you can't move? I say, move yourself in your mind. Dance in your dreams. It's the emotion that leads you to your next level of accomplishment. Ask God for help. If you have skepticism about God or your higher power, ask in your mind for help. Your prayers will be answered. It may show up in a friend's voice or through a stranger you meet on the street. It may come through something you read. The answers always show up. Just be opened to receive the possibility. Remember the cells of your body have the intelligence to heal. They repair themselves all the time. It is your responsibility to provide the proper environment so this can happen.

Take a walk in nature. Or sit outside. Watch how nature just happens. There is a life and death to everything. There is a rhythm to the way you "be." (There's that "beingness", again.) For me, I am finding my own internal rhythm through yoga. Aerobics didn't work for me. My body kept being thrown out of balance. Yoga put me more in touch with my internal self. I found out through yoga that my structural imbalance during aerobics kept throwing my pelvis out. I learned that it wasn't that I couldn't do aerobics, but it was the wrong form of exercise for my structural needs. I suddenly had more compassion and understanding for myself. What's important for me to bring out here is that the more I do yoga, the easier it is to breathe. It also allows me the ability to feel my scoliosis from the inside, and to send breath to areas that have been starved. I had always been led to believe by the doctors that I had some sort of malformation that needed help. Their way of helping me was to put me into a backbrace. (Stuffing my spirit into a small shoe, is how I view it now.) Unfortunately that time in my life left me with a huge emotional scar. Through yoga I have learned that my breath can transform anything. I had muscles that were weak and needed attention. How metaphoric our bodies can be. We all have strengths and weaknesses. I learned my body's structure is not who I am. It is only my vehicle while I am on this earth.

Another thing I like to do is go out into the woods and just lie down to watch the trees. (Or watch from a window.) I began noticing or contemplating how perfect the trees are. Some were twisted. Some were really bent. Some were tall and straight. There are even Siamese twin trees with one trunk. I felt like God was personally talking to me and telling me that we all are perfect. We all have what it takes to survive. We just have to be nourished properly. I grant you, some bodies are more pleasing to the eye than others, but beauty is in the eyes of the beholder. So, love yourself. You're all you got.

I found that seeking the wisdom that my body holds for me was a dramatic step to take. It leads you into emotions that you don't necessarily want to feel. Underneath this is another part of you just waiting to surface. Yoga helped me learn more about how my body had been operating. Without judgment, only compassion. Once you realize the magnificence of you and your body, the dance with self becomes more enjoyable. And another state of being is birthed.

Getting this energy moving allows you to move into a new state of consciousness. But getting energy to move is another thing. How do you do it if you don't have the drive to do it? I can answer that the only way I know how. First thing, don't beat yourself up over the idea. You might try to do it on a sunny day when you automatically feel more uplifted. Try walking, it's the easiest form of exercise. I know there were some days I couldn't get out of bed due to all my physical pain, but those were the days I tried my hardest to take just a small walk. Try and begin thinking about moving for only ten minutes. Just take baby steps. And when you feel up to it, put on some music and dance. Begin by just moving your fingers. Start adding your wrists. Your arms. Move up to your shoulders. Circle your head. Just feel the movements. Enjoy yourself. Breathe. Add a little hip action. Circle your hips. Add some movement from your feet. Before you know it, you have a little dance going on with yourself. You are moving energy. Take in some deep breaths. Relax your mind. Straighten your back, lift up your chest, "aliven" your spine. This is what it is like to awaken the body.

I know there is a lot of hype out there saying we need cardiovascular workouts. We're told body building should be done to prevent osteoporosis. There are a lot of things we are told we need. Your body will tell you what you need. Just ask it. As far as basics go, it needs water to help flush the debris and to replenish your cells with fluids. We need clean air to breathe. We need to pay attention to our diets. We need positive thoughts and to surround ourselves with uplifting people. This includes ridding your life of toxic people. You know the ones; those that drain your energy. Awakening the body awakens the mind and the emotions to a higher state of being. All these things are interrelated. Pretty neat, eh?

The water, air and food we eat is just the beginning to help bring our bodies into alignment with the new self that is emerging. Being mindful of how to get there is another thing. Meditation is very important. It is a necessity. Quiet moments for yourself to still the mind and listen to your breath is nourishment your soul is crying out for. When I first started to meditate, I would lie down and say, "Okay, I'm here. What do I need to do?" I didn't know about listening to my breath. I was a babe in new territory. What made the difference for me was my development as an artist. Who knew that underneath all that mind chatter was a talent ready to be expressed. As I lay silently on the floor, I began seeing pictures come into my thoughts. They were in geometric form. All I had to do was get myself some canvases and begin the process of producing. I was totally guided on how to use color. My inner artist was bursting out all over. It was so exciting! It was as if my soul was crying out with joy. In full color! I know it won't be like that for everyone, but that is how I began with my meditation practice. Like anything, with practice, you just get better. I look forward to starting my days with this silence. I like to begin my day fresh and alive.

I once read that you should do some type of strength exercise when you feel overwhelmed. I think that is great advice. Try using an exercise bike or jumping on a small trampoline. Or do a few push-ups. Anything to release that built up emotional pressure. When I feel uptight about something, I like to do stretching or some type of dance movement. It allows the denser energy to pass through more gracefully and helps you to regain your inner balance. It restores your natural breath. Remember that your breath is your balance. If you breathe shallow, your whole self will lack the quality of life it so desires. An imbalance could show up in some phase of your life whether, it manifests as a cold, as asthma, chronic back pain or even cancer. Your body is God's vehicle to talk to you. Awareness of your body is another bridge to help you begin your journey to blend your physical self with your spiritual self (also known as your God-self).

Listening to your body is sort of like body therapy. When you are irritable or tired, you might want to consider what you are eating. I have learned from my dog, Samantha, not to eat when emotionally upset. She's amazing to observe. As for myself, I know that I tend to eat out of frustration, looking for something sweet just to make myself feel better. Thank goodness I do not have a weight problem. What I have also noticed is that Samantha picks up on what is going on with Terry or me. She is very in tune with us. In her own way, she is probably telling us to watch how we eat and not to stuff ourselves. Our digestion can only do so much at one time. With all the impurities in our food and water, tripled by emotional stress, the digestion is often on overload. Just take it easy and begin listening to what your new "therapist" is telling you.

Another way I have tapped into myself and my body's needs is listening to my thoughts. If I become burdened with too many worries at one time, I take a break and breathe (there's that breath again). I breathe in real slowly and ask the universe to lift my burdens from me. Before I know it, my inner self seems calmer and more in sync with my surroundings. Again, I try to surround myself with positive people.

If we begin to learn how to tap into what our body is saying, we can begin to develop our intuition. Our intuition is the feeling we get in our gut. (That's why it is called gut feeling.) If you haven't been able to tap into your intuitive side, notice how your body is responding to its surroundings. For years, I bargained with my body in what I call my negotiation with God. I did this because I was unaware of energy and how God was talking to me. I had intuitive thoughts that would come through for me, but I was unaware of how to interpret them. For instance, in one of my jobs I kept re-creating and re-living my unresolved family "issues." You know the ones that follow you into your job and personal relationships. Every year my back problems would exacerbate until I was bed-ridden. Finally, after four years of this repetitive experience, I decided to tell my body if "it" (as if my body was separate from me) could make it one year without any flare-ups, I would quit my job. I really did believe that my problems were the result of my job and the stresses I had encountered with my extended family unit at work. One year passed and my body was doing fine. I really wanted to continue in this environment, because I hated looking for a new job. I was comfortable in my discomforts. Does this relate to you?

Anyway, a promise is a promise, and I needed to keep my promise to myself.

I quit my job and found a new one closer to my home. Within two weeks I got an awakening. I had jumped from the frying pan into the fire. This new job was a nightmare. I suddenly realized it was not my old job, but it was me. I didn't know what that meant. All I knew was that I needed to take a deeper look at myself. Yada, yada, yada...and my next step was in the direction of getting me out of that unhappy environment. That's when I moved to Atlanta. Why did I bring this story up in this part of my memoirs? It's because it was God who was talking to me through my body. And I am trying to awaken you to listen to your body.

Sometimes we don't know where to start because we become so overwhelmed as to what our next step is. When I moved to Charlotte, I got to explore the shadow side of myself. We all have this side. It feels like a dark cloud hanging over you. I asked God to help me through this. I was lucky because I had a game plan. We all need a game plan. I found myself unable to separate my unhappiness from my new home. I really thought it was just the wrong house, or that Charlotte was the wrong city. I was so used to having my body tell me when a situation was not in harmony with me, that I never questioned that God was awakening me to listen to another aspect of myself. My emotions were being awakened. And it was not pleasant. As it turns out, this house was the perfect house for me because it allowed me to innocently awaken to a new and higher level of communication with God. I was being enlightened to a new way of listening. And out of this communication, I found myself with a new game plan. I'll pass what I have learned on to you.

First, when stuck in pain in your physical body, look around at your surroundings. It's time for a physical move. It's time to reevaluate your "self" from the inside out. Find a place that resonates with you. VERY IMPORTANT! If a place (or person) doesn't make you feel good, it's not right for you. Our bodies will begin to shut down. When I moved to Atlanta, as soon as I got acclimated to my new environment, I loved it. It felt like home. Have you ever felt like this? Charlotte was a different story. I went to Charlotte with such a positive attitude. I knew that I needed to get my house situated to suit us. But that was so hard to do. Hard not in the physical sense but in the emotional sense. I found myself needing a new game plan.

Secondly, don't get yourself too overwhelmed. That's where I was. It took me seven months to begin to take the necessary steps to see if Charlotte was the problem, or if it was my home. I started with a couple of rooms in my house. The house is a wonderful metaphor for your body. The house did feel better. And I felt better emotionally. I thought we could now make Charlotte our home. I was given a new environment in which to find myself. Within one week I

KNEW. (There's that gut feeling, a "knowingness" that something is just not right.) **It was not me nor my home, but the energy that surrounded me.** The energy did not match my vibration. It was not bad, not good; not anything. I just did not resonate with the energy there. My soul was not being nourished. It was hard for me to grasp because I did not have knowledge or understanding of what I was experiencing. I felt like I was suspended in life, like I was just existing. Even scarier, I felt like I was in a holding pattern with a magnifying glass looking back onto my life.

On one hand, it was interesting; and on the other, it was very scary. I was filled with so many emotions. Looking back, I know I was doing work directed from a higher place. I was not only healing my own past, present and future, I was helping to uplift my surrounding area. What I am trying to impress upon you is to work on raising your consciousness. Do your work. Don't stand still. You may feel you don't have anything to work on, but you probably do. If you like the way you are, and don't feel you need to change, look at how your relationships are doing. Consider your family and your job. Listen to the words that come out of your mouth about others and yourself. Then you'll know…and get to work!

Lastly, learn to separate what is yours and not yours. Learn to set some positive boundaries for yourself. Sometimes it helps to take a break. Look for a place in which to take refuge. Give yourself the gift of vacationing in the mountains or at the beach. These are healing places. Try and do it alone. It would be great if you could give yourself at least a few weeks in this new environment. Then, when you reintroduce yourself into your old environment, you'll immediately "feel" if it still works for you. If you take the time to listen, your body will speak to you in a voice that is loud and clear. If getting away is not feasible, get yourself reconnected to nature in some other way. Your body will talk loud and very clear.

I hope I have raised some valuable questions in your mind. We are here on earth raising planetary consciousness by bringing peace and love to earth. Peace starts when you bring it towards yourself first. It will be a win-win situation for all those that choose to participate in life with you. After all, we all want the same thing; LOVE!

Food for thought: How many of you applaud yourself for a job well done? I do it all the time. I especially do it for my body. I congratulate mine for the elimination process it does so beautifully. We tend to take our bodies for granted, and I think they need praise. Our elimination process is the only way we can rid our internal self from toxins. Our bodies are magnificent. Why not bless it and give thanks for the job it does so well. And if you are one of those people that don't move regularly (you know what I mean) find a natural way to do it. Get yourself regulated. You may not be giving your body the time to do it. It does not like to be rushed. I know sometimes when I am traveling, I feel rushed before I leave. I tell my body to get prepared. This will be the only chance it has to "move" for the next few hours. Surprisingly enough, it responds to my wishes.

If you have a hard time listening to your body, seek out someone who can assist and teach you HOW to interpret the messages. Just like sports trainers, there are spiritual coaches too. Spiritual coaching is a new field in psychic attunement (also known as intuitive abilities). As we continue blending Eastern and Western medicines, there will be more and more coaching available. Your body will give you its best if you give it your best. Seek the knowledge it desires, and feed your soul for internal health.

One thing I forgot to mention. We are human beings. (Duh!) We survive best with the touch from others. If we eliminate human touch from our menu, our lives will suffer as a result. When I first got married, it was very important to have hug therapy. That's what we called it. On our hurried days, hugs are a necessity. Remember, water, food, exercise, rest/meditation, hugs and sunlight. That's a pretty full diet to well-being. Fill your days with being well. (There's that word again.) Dance with the sunlight. Stroll with the moon. Play with the air. These are all ways of getting in touch with your body, which elevates your state of "being."

I hope I have gracefully added some colorful ways to get to know your body, and to help blend it with ways of being. Be creative. Have fun! Enjoy yourself!

Blending My Two Worlds

*I*t's not easy to blend the two worlds that make up the whole package of self. The emotional, mental, and physical has to be balanced with the spiritual. We are blessed with our physical bodies, and God is working through us as spirit. In essence, God is having a human experience through us. For those that find that hard to believe, play with it. Test yourself. Think a thought. Watch it unfold. If you think a negative thought, it will manifest. If you think a positive thought, it will manifest. The more you become aware of your thoughts, the more you will see God in action. Carolyn and I both say if we had not connected ourselves with God and allowed Him to work through us, we would still be where we were. We may have gotten a little better, but not much. Since Carolyn's near death experience, we both have been gifted with extraordinary senses. We are able to enable others to be set free from their pains and woes. We don't exactly know how we do it. All we know is that by being in our presence, and stating our intentions, allows the seeker to be lifted to a new level of consciousness. The seeker is then gifted to begin to seek more. It is their choice. That's where free choice comes in. As I move through each day, I love to watch this unfold. It is the extra sight I have been given. I have been asked if we are healers. Are we mystics? I do not know. I/we just know that we are walking this earth with more enjoyment. We are here as teachers, teaching those we come in contact with another way of being.

Carolyn and I are not above life's challenges. We still have our own dramas to deal with. The only difference is we have tools to work with, and angels and guides to help lead us in a more suitable direction. If the struggle persists, we ask for new guides to help assist us to a more desirable state of mind. I am constantly pushing my mind and body past its limits. It's who I am. I am that woman who seeks to unveil the mysteries of life and to bless and praise the miracles all around me. I re-create and re-invent myself all the time. I throw out old habits, old lifestyles that no longer suit me. It's no different than spring-cleaning.

The ultimate goal I have for each day is happiness. I feel the toughest daily lesson for me is to stay on the path of positive thinking. Our thinking process is so powerful and is conditioned to past negative misinformation. I try to stay conscious of the communication I am sending myself. One bad thought can lead you to another, and, "whoops," you can be on that dark and narrow road the whole day. Do you ever find yourself in doomsville? Sit quietly and begin listening to your thoughts. It may be necessary to just go back to bed and start over. The key to help keep your spirits uplifted is to keep out the negative thoughts that bring about negative effects. This includes the people I call "toxic." You know the ones. Start eliminating them from your life.

When a negative thought presents itself, and you accept it (i.e. I am not worthy) the physical can take over. You are caught in a negative downward spiral. That is why negative talking is so draining. I have been guilty on many occasions of participating amongst co-workers or family members, and the results are always the same. I feel exhausted, drained and angry. It has become my conscious effort to no longer participate in such conversations. If you find yourself bombarded within a negative conversation, the thing to do is instantly excuse yourself from the conversation, and do not accept it as truth. God speaks the truth. Love is truth and anything other than love is false truth. Learn to slam that door shut immediately because you do not want any negative thought forms attached to you. Remember these thoughts are not of your soul and spirit. Refocus on what is real for you and gear your thoughts in that direction.

I am not going to say that this is easy. I find myself constantly putting myself back on the right path. Our thoughts need to be monitored at all times.

As I look back over my time spent in Charlotte, I was healing from the wounds inflicted by negative self-talk and the negative influences in my life. I was even purging out old complaints. I recognized they weren't all mine. Being a twin, I have learned to identify the ones that are of my own making. These negative emotions were stuck in my physical form. I was getting my much-needed mental and emotional realignment.

Life is a balancing act. We have to be physically, mentally, emotionally and spiritually in balance. When any part of us is outweighed, unhappiness manifests. Unfortunately, I grew up in a family that did not know how to nurture each other. So this is a huge challenge for me to overcome. I also have this tendency to want to withdraw and not participate because it is my method of self-protection. I have to keep reminding myself to get out there and be a participant. Share myself. Make someone smile. After all, being an ex-hygienist, it's still part of my job to make someone's smile be brighter.

Dreams... a form of healing

Dreams can help us find our deepest, darkest secrets. Dreams can also subconsciously reveal what we would like to create in our own lives. But we can only make these desires and dreams come true with a real "game plan." Dreams can also warn us when we are in danger. Dreams don't always occur while we are asleep. Dreams are a different state of consciousness. Dreams can actually transport you to places your body cannot take you. (This is very important in the healing process.) Dreams can get you "unstuck" from life's challenges. Dreams can be what you write about. Start writing. Start journaling. " Dream up" what you want to see happening in your own life. After all, you are the main character in your life's drama. You can write a very happy ending.

I call this the dream journaling of "living happily-ever-after." Allow yourself the luxury to dream. If you have forgotten how, just lie quietly. Put on some soft and soothing music and allow your mind to drift off to never-never-land. Begin by breathing deeply. See what comes to you. If your intention is stated beforehand, it will be easier to bring your creation to light. It is really no different than having an idea pop into your mind, except this time you are focusing your energies on creating happiness. Enjoy the process!

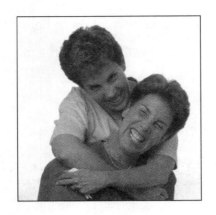

Is The Grass Greener on the Other Side?

Families

Families, let's face it, sometimes they're hard. I have often felt that I was let go to find my own way. Yes, it was painful, but out of pain came my growth, and I wouldn't trade my life for anyone else's. I'll make this statement now, before I go off on a writing tangent. I had always thought that the worst of my pain and sorrow had stemmed from my family. As I was thinking that thought one day, I suddenly realized that it was not true. The cause of my pain and sorrow has been me standing in the way of myself. Not allowing my inner voice to be expressed was one of the ways that I stifled myself. I say this now, because as I write about my family, I have a whole different perspective.

Is the grass always greener on the other side? I don't think so. There are so many types of families today, such as stepfamilies, single-mom families, you name it, and we're experiencing it. I think that growing up, we thought families should be stereotyped as June and Ward Cleaver. In my case this did not happen. (Television is so impressionable on young minds, isn't it?)

I could get angry and blame my father for not doing a better job as both mother and father. I felt that way for most of my life. The outcome was always the same…a lot of heartache. What I needed to learn was how to forgive him. This was a very hard lesson, because I allowed myself to keep getting caught in the negative emotion of blame. That only kept the negative emotions alive, and kept me very stuck.

I finally had to step aside and ask myself, "What do I want to accomplish right now?" I wanted harmony and peace of mind. The only way I was going to get what I desired was to forgive. I needed first to forgive myself for keeping these negative emotions alive so that I could finally just let them go.

I knew that this "project" was much bigger than I was, and I had to turn it over to my higher power. I had to ask God to forgive me, and I had to ask my father to forgive me. I then asked God for an attitude adjustment, and once again it was time to move on.

This is where my writing has taken me. I was desperately in need of an "attitude adjustment," but that wasn't all. Do you ever ask for an attitude adjustment? If the answer is "no," give it a try. I needed to get off the path of negative thinking and quit harping on things that either didn't happen, or should have happened, or could have happened. To put it bluntly, I needed to "get over it." I needed a higher perspective.

We are born into our families, but that is not all there is to it. I said before that I never felt like I fit into my family; but from God's perspective, it was the perfect family for me. Through my own learning, I now believe that we **choose** our family and our life lessons. In retrospect, it was the perfect family in which both Carolyn and I could grow in consciousness as a team.

There are different "levels of consciousness" in each family, just like there are different grade levels in school, on up to college and graduate school. I really feel that Carolyn and I have been together for a very long time, and not just in this lifetime. We both feel that I have had more "earth years" than Carolyn, yet Carolyn is more evolved spiritually than I. This is neither good nor bad, nor is one better than the other; but it is the perfect blend for two souls that come together to grow. We are each other's teachers. We are here sharing our knowledge with one another. I believe this is why we were born into our family. We are here to teach our family how to share. We are here learning our own lessons of love.

God's lessons are simple. Allow yourself to reach for your truths to uncover the real you. Allow yourself to learn how to accept your family, to learn discernment, to find or develop your own integrity, to forgive, to accept rejection and move on. God wants each of us to know he loves us. God's definition of love is different than what we have been taught. Children already know that love "just is." Love has no strings attached to it. We as adults teach them to forget their true essence.

Unfortunately, as we grow up, love begins to take on a conditional definition. These become our veils, the protective barriers and boundaries we place around ourselves. Sometimes when you think of yourself as a grain of sand within the Universe, you can easily become overwhelmed and feel unimportant. But the true reality is, if you come back into your own world and connect with your magnificence, you will notice you do make a difference. I don't think that there is one person on this planet that has not been influenced by his or her family's beliefs and behaviors about how love is expressed and communicated.

God wants us to know love is just love. It is energy. You cannot buy it; it is not something you own. You can try to express it, but that always comes with a slew of other emotions that get muffled in the translation. Love is not simply three little words, expressed as "I love you." As humans we think that is love, but it is much more. Love is the highest of all vibrations, and we all are in pursuit of it. It is a vibration that no one can teach you how to feel. It's something we must each work towards individually. It's learning how to open your heart, remove your veils and rediscover the real you that lies dormant deep inside.

Learning to love yourself comes with sloughing off the old ideas that you have about yourself. The way in which you see yourself is not the way that others see you. The hardest part for me is that each time I come in contact with my family, I immediately find myself regressing into my old patterns. That is not uncommon, because our families see us in a certain light. What I found myself thinking was that all of the work I had done on myself had been wasted. Or, worse, maybe it wasn't real. I have to hurry and slam that door shut to negative thinking before the negativity begins having a voice all its own. I have to remember that I have grown by leaps and bounds. I have to remember old behaviors and personality traits have been stirred up. I find I become the person I am striving not to be. I have to recognize it is part of me and I need to accept and possibly use that "old me" as a gauge on how far I have come. I have to remember that not every member of my family has been working on himself or herself, or even sees a need to do so. I have to recognize that my father and my other sisters are doing the same thing that Carolyn and I are doing—growing in soul consciousness. The difference between Carolyn and me and the rest of the family is the level and degree of our consciousness.

No family is perfect. I cough a little with that thought in mind. I guess that is why it is called "tough love." Some families are harder to be around than others. I realize that some families do get along. I have learned that one's "personality" is not the sum total of who one is. It is part of one's "outer mask," and buried deep underneath that armor of personality is a real person, reaching out to be loved. I am now able to recognize the "God-essence" of each person. However, that discovery is not really for me to make; it is for each person to re-discover whom he or she is. I know that deep underneath each person's wounds, there's a child of God, just waiting to be loved. I can do that. That is easy. It is being around the different "personalities" that is not so easy.

One of the lessons I have learned is to pray that each person finds his or her own way to the God within, and that I accept where they currently are. I do this everyday. I feel that it's my job to ask God for His assistance when I see someone struggling. If I do nothing else, I must get out of the way and watch His works unfold. It's not up to me to want to hurry the process along, because opening one's heart to God is always in God's time, and not one second before.

When I think about how very blessed Carolyn and I have been, I sigh with a huge smile on my face and a feeling of deep appreciation in my heart. We have the gift to see our spiritual evolution taking place. It's not always a pleasant experience, but there is always a positive ripple affect. The more work that Carolyn and I do on us, the more our family is affected. At times, we still get blamed for creating disharmony. In my heart we are not really to blame; it is just the process that we are going through as a family unit to get to the love that is buried deep inside each one of us.

I feel that sometimes my sisters may be judging Carolyn and me for what they perceive to be hypocrisy, because if we were so God-like, why would we still react in the old ways? I do not claim I am above all of this. I still have my own stuff to go through, and will for as long as I live. What I have realized is that if I take a deep breath before reacting in a situation, I do much better. Deep breathing is very important, and always seems to help clear my mind and relax my body.

What it does mean is we are relating to family members in a way that is familiar and comfortable. We respond to each other as we did as kids. If I didn't know better, this sounds like a catch twenty-two. Could we all be a big giant mirror reflecting into the other's behavior what needs attention?

I try to keep in mind that I am learning to separate myself from my old behaviors and the way that my family sees me. I find that I am always in a lesson; trying to master how to relate to others in a more loving way. Notice the vibration you're sending out: Are you sending "vibes" that are kind and gentle to others? Because what you send out to others is exactly what you get back. Once again this is the lesson of cause and effect.

Where am I going with all of this? I would like to arouse some curiosity in your minds. I would like you to begin to question yourself. What is God trying to awaken in you? What does He want from you? First of all, communication with God must become a two-way street. (Communication with anyone has to be a two-way street.) Ask and you shall receive, but first give yourself the permission to receive. God wants you to know yourself. It is vital to learn to reach out and really ask for His help. Acknowledge Him in your times of joy by giving thanks. Work to bring peace of mind and heart to yourself. Open up to the happiness, joy and gladness that is already inside you. Stop judging yourself. Judgment has a negative response. Placing judgment upon others is a mirror back to you on HOW critical you are to yourself. As you open up this communication, you will see that God is working through you, by creating miracles all around you. That is part of the "Is-ness."

One of my favorite television shows is "Touched by an Angel." It's a great family show. It's so real. Watching their episodes is a great way of learning how special you really are.

I could have gone back and been real nitpicky about my family, but the irony is that they were the ones who allowed me to grow most rapidly. Yes, there has been a lot of disharmony within our family, and no, I don't like it, BUT that was the catalyst for me to create something better for myself. I wanted and searched for more peace in my life and now I am getting it. I have healed my emotional wounds by creating a loving and kind family with my husband, Terry, and dog, Samantha. That is my family. There is finally peace in my heart. I have a new foundation of what I want to feel like.

I have also created an extended family with two girls who lost their mother. We now call ourselves "inherited mother and daughters." I had always joked about wanting two girls, in their twenties, to have as daughters. I never dreamed that this would become my reality. Maybe I missed a step by not becoming a birthmom, but God always answers my prayers. It is time for me to learn lessons with my new extended family. I can serve as a friend who has been there with an open heart to help them along their way. I am grateful to Amy and Nicole for helping me achieve another level of growth. There will probably always be sadness in our hearts for not having natural birthmoms to grow and share our lives with; but the miracle we have with each other is our opportunity to share our lives and hearts with the replacement God has provided us. Hopefully I can make their journeys through life a little less painful.

I want to acknowledge the family I do have. I must remember that my parents were my ticket to this school called earth and that they, too, are in that school. My sisters were the catalysts that helped me grow. We are ALL here on earth to learn to feel, deal, and heal our emotions.

Through my sharing of how I "used" my family dynamics to help me grow, I hope that I have raised questions in your mind about the "what ifs" of life. If you think you don't have to work on yourself, I'd like to challenge you to rethink that statement. If you don't think that you have an effect on your family, I'd like to challenge you to look at how well your relationships are doing. We all live in the same pond (meaning-our families, our environment, and the world), and when a rock is thrown into that pond, it causes ripples. Each one of us is affected whether we are aware of it or not. I'd also like to challenge you to impact your family in a positive way, to let go of your old ways of relating. Look for new opportunities as to how you can behave. We can make a difference on this planet, one by one, we can lead in love.

Carolyn and I joke with each other about dragging the other one around. Our dance step was TWO BY TWO. As we began to separate and get in touch with God, one by one, our dance step changed and we became more harmonious with our inner selves. Being a twin is probably one of the hardest lessons you can have in life. It is learning to take responsibility for the things that need to change. It is like looking at yourself and having life reflect into you what needs attention. Being a singleton, you don't have that luxury of seeing yourself. Being a twin has provided a deep learning about loving and accepting oneself...all of me, including that extended part of myself. We did get it! We hope you will get it, too.

The Truth of the Matter is

*U*ntying my knots was not just me untying from Carolyn and the family dysfunctions that no longer worked; it was about discovering and unfolding my life's patterns. It was about me forming a new pattern of how I want to live my life now. I have a new future awaiting me, and I must let go of my past. I want to surround myself with truth.

It seems that family members are the most critical of us and yet the most truthful. But do we ever tell the truth, I mean the real truth, to each other and to ourselves? Was I really truthful to Carolyn? To myself? Growth through truth hurts, but is it any more painful than staying stuck in the destructive dynamics of dysfunction? I needed to change my feelings of frustration about writing this book with Carolyn. The core essence of our journey was very similar, but the ingredients that both of us wanted to put into the book were different. I had been waiting for Carolyn to lead me out of this project and into the next one. I wanted Carolyn to come along with me in my career as a writer. What I needed to do was ask her some questions. I asked her point blank if she had any desire to write her own book. She had so much knowledge that I did not have. She matter-of-factly stated, "No way. You're the writer." After that comment, I took a deep breath and knew what I needed to do. I needed to separate myself even further from her. Our paths had taken a turn in different directions. I knew I needed to finish this book by myself. My gut always knew this, but I was scared to let her go. I was scared to move on without her, and yet my soul's desire was to write with full expression. I knew my soul was going to win. All I had to do was let go and let God lead me into my most difficult role. That role was about to unfold for me.

Heart to Heart

What my family never knew about Carolyn and me was that although we were always together, it was not always comfortable. As one grows more in love (remember it is a vibration), one must start discarding the negatives from one's life. In my heart I was still in search for a better relationship with Carolyn. I just didn't know how to get there. I didn't have the right words to say to her. But as life has it, change was inevitable. I knew our relationship was not as harmonious as I had wanted it to be. I had really wanted to tell Carolyn what was in my heart for many, many years, but I felt speechless. I felt unequipped to handle the possibility of rejection from her. I didn't want her to feel I was rejecting her either. Everytime I wanted to say what was really on my mind, I fell short, always stuffing the words back into my psyche. I knew that she would just take them as being critical and hurtful, and that would not be my intention at all. Our sisterly squabbles would continue as always. What I didn't know at the time, as I was having this conversation in counseling, was that Carolyn, at the same time, was sitting down to write what was in her heart that she was unable to say to me! Through writing, one eliminates the outer voice of confusion and lets the inner voice from the heart be heard. Our writing allowed us to move to our next step of communication, peacefully. I highly recommend this "letter writing." It's a great way to open doors of communication and let loved ones know your heart.

(Interestingly enough, with this shift in our communication, the Universe helped put us back on our shared path as writers.)

Forgiveness

*F*orgiveness plays a huge part in one's healing process. When you forgive someone, you are setting in motion the release of an emotional debt. It's like wiping the slate clean for both parties involved. There are so many elements in the forgiveness process. The first step is an action step, like placing a call or writing a letter. I think for myself this process was a little different. I had been working so hard on finding compassion and understanding for the people who had not been kind or loving to me, that I kept blame in the subconscious part of my mind. This blame kept me in a vicious cycle from which I so desperately needed to free myself.

What I had to learn was that it was really the act of giving to myself that would set me free. FOR: GIVE-no name attached. At a very subtle level Carolyn and I kept blaming each other for even the smallest incident. This blaming only kept our tension fueled. Have you ever experienced tension with someone, but couldn't figure out a reason for it? Unfortunately, my family had a history of treating each other in this manner. It took a conscious effort on my part for me to uncover behaviors that no longer suited me. I learn that the conflict I continued creating with Carolyn was a battle that was self-serving.

This was one of the ugly ones. This vicious battle of "right" or "wrong" put both of us on the defensive. It was "I" who needed to make this conscious behavior change in order to stop this non-verbal argument before it got started. I was enabling myself to move in the direction that my soul had been directing me. I was re-aligning my heart with truth and integrity. I wanted to be surrounded by more love. This was the best gift I could give myself. Carolyn and I were reflecting into the other one what needed attention, and it was my desire to shine brightly.

I needed to forgive myself for all the wasted moments, but more importantly, I needed to applaud myself for finally getting it. I needed to have the compassion for myself and the wisdom to know that all my sorrows, angers, frustrations and grief have been the lessons I was put on earth to learn.

It doesn't matter how conscious one becomes; we will always have lessons to learn. There are lessons on how to treat the body, and how to love the body. All physical ailments fall into this category. God is so magnificent, because in order to get to the physical lessons, you still have to go through the emotional and mental ones. When you can reach a harmonious blend of knowing what is in your heart and learning to live with love, the spiritual realm of consciousness will translate this as "heaven on earth." Life is eternity. Wouldn't it be more fun to live forever with love all around you?

Sounds easy, but the catch twenty-two, again, is that love is a vibration. Not everyone is comfortable in that vibration. Or let's say that another way. Not everyone is familiar with that vibration. Picture love like a piano and imagine the keyboard. One note leads to another in harmony. You move through one key at a time, one note at a time- one lesson at a time. Opening up to this vibration is a process. When you are being overwhelmed in a physical, emotional or mental crisis, it is time to recognize that you are in front of a spiritual door just waiting to be opened. Your spirit is reaching out to help you. You just have to reach back and ask God/Spirit to help bring light to your pains.

Loving, healing, feeling and forgiveness are processes. In my own healing, and with the healing of my family relationships, sometimes all I have to do is ask God to intervene and take care of the details. I'll just show up and do my work. That is all that is expected of me, and in my heart I know I have done my best.

In the Final Hour

After years of writing, it suddenly dawned on me to ask God what message He wanted me to deliver. A picture came to my mind. It was me awakening my body from shoulders turned inward to the expansion of my chest. I felt as if I was a flowering tulip awakening from a deep, winter sleep. As I awakened, I heard a faint voice inside my head whisper the words, "Grow your heart." I feel I have done just that.

With the conclusion of our book, we challenge you to ask yourself if you are truly happy in your relationship with self. Are all aspects of your life being fulfilled? If not, what can you do about it? Are you willing to go the extra mile for yourself to find out? You are the deliberate creator of how well you will be.

Carolyn and I have been very lucky to have each other to simultaneously walk down this road together. We have recognized that we are two individuals walking two different paths that are interwoven beautifully by the Divine. We want you to know that what we have been experiencing doesn't just relate to twins. As mentioned earlier, these inter-relationships can be between mother and daughter, father and son, husband and wife, between friends and even with someone deceased. The point we have been trying to bring forward is to recognize where your "stuckness" lies so you can let go and bring about other possibilities. There is no limit to how much joy we can create for ourselves. Yes, I have finally awakened my heart to live life as if it was my final hour. I have begun healing my family relationships to the best of my ability. The relationship with Natalie has taken a sudden shift, and I actually enjoy being around her. In my growing, learning and allowing the other person to be who they are, I have provided myself with the gift of enjoyment. It is what I have longed for but didn't know how to obtain. In my relationships with Nicole and Amy, I have surrendered to allowing them to be in my life. This was divinely orchestrated from above. My dad and I have let down a lot of our guards. I am seeing him as a person, with all his faults, and have released him from the pedestal that I placed him on as a child. (After all, he is only human.) Debra, the sister that didn't like my tone, has taught me another way of being. She has taught me to be softer--in her own little way, and for that I am grateful. Carolyn and I have let go of our co-dependency with each other and have begun blending into a more harmonious "couple." We are no longer trying to be "all" for the other one. We have set each other free (as much as possible, being a twin).

In a waking dream, I finally "got" what Norman Cousins was saying to me that day. He wanted me to "write first and then speak." It suddenly dawned on me, I was a piece of his puzzle. He was one of the forerunners on how the mind/body connection affects our immune system. He believed in laughter. He felt that it was laughter that healed him during his most critical times. He believed life was an adventure in learning how to forgive. I get a little picture in my head right now of him saying, "Lighten up down there. You're too serious." The piece of knowledge I began sharing with him that day was how the spirit connects to heal the physical body. As Carolyn and I have said before, and this needs to be repeated; if it wasn't for our spiritual reconnection to God, we wouldn't have made it through our physical crises. Our reconnecting to God, and allowing Him to just take over, was nothing short of a miracle. I was looking to Dr. Cousins to help me to my next step but, in reality, I already had the information. Information is knowledge. And knowledge is power. The question became, what was I going to do with this information. Life really is simple. Grow in wisdom and let the love in. Show up and be present. We, as humans, get so caught up in the materialistic world we have forgotten what is real. God is our dancing partner and you, too, can dance two by two.

I guess you can tell by now that I, Marilyn, have been the main voice in our book. We both couldn't talk at the same time; it's a twin-thing. So, lastly, but not forgotten, **Carolyn returns in her own voice.**

So what have I learned while on this journey?

I've learned that life is our school, full of lots and lots of lessons. Life itself is the journey.

I've learned you keep on learning.

I've learned that family and its dynamics spur you into your lessons. I found it was the greatest way to learn and grow in my Soul.

I've learned from being a twin that I am unique (and I bless this). Even though mirrors can be painful, if you look at yourself closely you can find your "pot of gold." Being a twin has allowed me to learn to communicate on a very different level that most singletons never get to experience. Being a twin has taught me, and continues to teach me, how to master relating to me...in accepting me.

I've learned through my mother's death that she gave me the greatest gift a mother can give. She gave me birth, and then by getting out of the way, by letting "totally" go of my reality, she allowed and enabled me to grow at a depth that I didn't even know existed.

I've learned from Roberta how to give your all and be your best in a relationship. I've learned that you make people feel "special" by showing them that you care. My father's divorce from Roberta allowed me to begin to open the buried wounds from my mother's death. Through their divorce, my grieving process began at a deeper level. It started me on my inward journey and my quest for wanting to know more about my purpose in this world. It was their separation that began my delving into "What life's all about."

I learned that being depressed with suicidal thoughts was my way of crying for help. The depression was the way I handled my guilt for wanting Mother to die. It was the way I punished myself for having these feelings. My suicidal thoughts were the result of the pain from these overwhelming feelings boiling inside of me. It was the way I pushed people away so they wouldn't see how much pain I was in. Depression was the behavior I chose to protect me from the outside world.

I've learned from dad's third marriage that realities/perceptions can change very quickly. Through their union, I was given the severe push I needed to leave the comfort zone of home. It shoved me to give up a foundation that no longer served me. Because of their union, I am truly thankful. Their marriage has taught me, and continues to teach me, to respect each person's path. I've learned not to get caught up in other people's lives…it is their life.

I've learned that Natalie's acting out towards me, towards Marilyn, was the way she handled her pain of feeling unwanted, unloved by Mother. I have learned through Natalie to let things roll off my back and not to take my life so seriously. I have learned that she is there for her family and friends. Even though she handles situations differently than I would, and she seems a little rough around the edges when talking with me…she is a true diamond.

I've learned that Debra's distancing from her sisters was the way she protected herself from feeling her pain and loss. I learned that her rejection of me was to protect herself from getting hurt by the ones she loved. As she kept herself separate from her family and me, it helped her draw from her internal resources to develop strength and endurance.

I've learned through having learning disabilities that there are different ways to learn. I learned to teach myself. I learned to call upon and use different angles when solving conflicts and problems. Having learning disabilities taught me to be creative. Learning disabilities taught me to push myself against all odds, despite feeling I couldn't do it, or that I didn't understand. The hardships I had in learning helped me develop the tools and a foundation that

I would later need in my life when I had my life-threatening illness. It taught me to keep searching and to never give up. It taught me perseverance.

I've learned from my father to stand on my own two feet. He taught me I didn't have to make it right for anyone else, he encouraged me to believe in myself, to be honest, to give from the heart. He taught me there is someone for everyone. He showed me money couldn't buy happiness. He pushed me to find my own way, my own home. I did. Home is where the heart is, and you can take that anywhere.

I have learned from having a life-threatening illness not to take a diagnosis as a final diagnosis—that there had to be a cause for me being so "reactive." I learned that even though I thought I had dealt with my mother's death intellectually and emotionally, my spirit was still wounded. Tapping into my spiritual component allowed me to have a complete healing. I learned that my mind, body and spirit are all connected. I learned that my body does talk to me and it will tell me what I need to know. I learned to listen to my body and to honor it. I learned to quiet my mind so I could hear the small voice within that guides me.

My near-death experience (NDE) allowed me to feel a deep peacefulness that I had never before experienced. I learned through the NDE that I had been a walking NDE all my life. I learned that you don't have to "almost" die in order to experience one. I learned that if you aren't living life to the fullest- with joy, with peace, with happiness- that you can get swallowed up in the fears that keep you stuck in your life. I call this entrapment. This experience allowed me to tap into my multi-dimensional self. I got a glimpse that there is more to life than what we see in our own reality. I learned we are more than our five senses. I learned there is a greater plan to all this "madness." As I returned to my body, I brought back glimpses of this plan. I now see life on a grander scale. One of the glimpses showed me I had to die in order to let go of all the guilt and grief I was carrying about my mom's death. It allowed me to forgive myself and to go on living. I now feel I see through magnifying glasses, on many different levels all at once. I'm not afraid of this because I've learned to work with these abilities, these gifts. By being present in this reality, I am able to work with unseen energies and to help others resolve conflicts in their souls. I am very blessed and honored to be of such service.

As a healer, I believe everyone can access his or her own abilities that lie within. I've learned to step aside and let the work flow through me. I've learned I cannot help everyone. I've learned I am damn good at my work. I've learned to empower myself and to empower others. I teach that if I can do this, so can you!

About relationships in general. I have learned that there are both good and unhealthy relationships in all aspects of your life, whether they are family, spouses, or co-workers. I've learned to let go of the unhealthy ones. I've learned I can't make relationships work unless both parties want to contribute. I've learned I don't have to make relationships right in order to keep what seems to be "harmony" within a family, within the job. I've learned I cannot make someone else happy. I've learned it is the responsibility of each person to create their own reality. If they choose to be unhappy, that is their choice. If they choose to be happy, that's GREAT. I've learned to let go of guilt. I've learned to forgive others and myself. I've learned not to blame. I've learned the biggest relationship I have is with myself. As I continue to learn to love me, to accept me, then I have more room for letting love in. I've learned to speak my truths and to take the baby steps I need when moving through "old" situations into a new way of being. I've learned to smile and praise me. I've learned through relationships that I have the power from within to change anything that makes me unhappy. I've learned through relationships that I am strong and I won't break.

Co-writing this book has taught me that everyone grieves differently. Everyone heals in his or her own time. As I was healing, I watched Marilyn heal too. I saw that we healed in different ways; that what was important to me in my healing process was not necessarily her "ah ha," and vice-versa. By co-authoring this book, it has helped me heal the wounds that were stuck in my psyche. Writing this book has set me free!

PART III

A Quick Summary

To tie this book together, Carolyn and I have decided to briefly list the high points of what we have learned. We consider ourselves very lucky to have had our wake-up calls and to be walking this path together.

- Connect to the spiritual side of yourself.
- *Seek more truth.*
- Pray a lot.
- *Open your heart to receive more love.*
- Let down your guards.
- *Develop your intuition.*
- Know there is more to life than what you see.
- *Learn to listen to your body.*
- Play with colors. Let colors enhance your mood.
- *Feed your mind with positive thoughts.*
- Nourish your body with high vibrational foods and drink a lot of pure, clean water.
- *Eliminate toxic people and things from your life.*
- Explore the energies of the plants and animals that are around you.

- *Develop, feed and nurture your relationships.*

- Walk your talk.

- *Learn to quiet your mind.*

- Meditate.

- *Keep a journal, or better still, write your own life's journey.*

- Seek harmony in your life.

- *Awaken yourself to your angels and guides. They're just waiting for you to ask them to help you.*

- Plant flowers, they're God's forms of laughter down here. Recognize you are one of those flowers.

- *Discard old habits, beliefs and behaviors that no longer suit you.*

- Remember, life's a dance, get yourself moving.

- *Reach for the stars and become one.*

- Dream big.

- *Trust your heart.*

- And finally, know God is holding your hand with each step that you take.

Recommended Reading

There are so many books out there just waiting to help you move into
a new point of reference for a better state of being. It is your job to find the
book(s) that resonate with you and help you continue to grow. Growing in
consciousness is feeding your soul. Your soul will always win. Below, we have
listed some books and a tape that have helped service our needs in reaching a
higher consciousness.

Many Lives, Many Masters—
Messages From The Masters—
Dr. Brian Weiss
Head First- The Biology of Hope—
Norman Cousins
You Can Have It All—
Arnold Patent
The Seat of the Soul—
Gary Zukav
Living in the Light—
Shakti Gawain

Return To Love—

Marianne Williamson

Motherless Daughters—

Hope Edelman

Dancing Naked in Front of the Fridge—

Nancy and Janna Sipes

The Artist's Way—

Julia Cameron

Love, Medicine and Miracles—

Bernie Siegel

Chicken Soup for the Soul—

Jack Canfield and Mark Victor Hansen

Angel Therapy—

Losing Pounds of Pain

Doreen Virtue

You Can Be Happy No Matter What—

Richard Carlson

Recommended Listening

Higher Ground—

Barbra Streisand

Workshops and Events

To Contact:

Marilyn and Carolyn are available for talks, lectures, and retreats. They also do private sessions, as well as long distant phone consultations. To contact Marilyn Segal or Carolyn Cohen:

TWIN-LYNN INC.
5579 B Chamblee Dunwoody Road
No. 139
Atlanta, Georgia 30338
e-mail: twin-lynn@mindspring.com
fax: 770-777-9441

Marilyn Segal

After 27 years of physical pain from a severe back injury and scoliosis, she experienced a dramatic, instantaneous healing. As a result of this experience she has devoted her life to understanding how the healing process works and teaching it to others. Marilyn practiced dental hygiene for 16 years and received a B.S. Degree in Health Science from East Tennessee State University. Marilyn is in training for certification in Consegrity Therapy from the Center of Energy Medicine in Wichita, Kansas.

Carolyn Cohen

As a gifted healer and survivor of a near-death experience, she is committed to guiding others to know and use the powerful energy within. Carolyn has her masters in counseling from East Tennessee State University and a postgraduate degree in Allied Health from Emory University.

They were featured in a segment in the TBS documentary, **The Heart of Healing.** Both currently work privately with clients and do phone consultations. They have been studying energy medicine for ten years. Carolyn and Marilyn reside in Atlanta with their husbands and dogs.

Order Form

Title:	Price	Qty.	Amt.
Whose Illness Is It Anyway? A spirtual journey to wellness	$16.95		
The Heart Speaks by Marilyn A delightful motivational and inspirational book about healing.	$11.95		
Precious Reflections by Carolyn Spiritual reflections that bring you back to the moment.	$10.95		
Subtotal:			
S & H $3.95 first book .95 each additional			
Tax: 7% for GA **Total:**			

Please send check or money order to:

Twin-Lynn, Inc.
5579 B Chamblee Dunwoody Rd.
No. 139
Atlanta, GA 30338